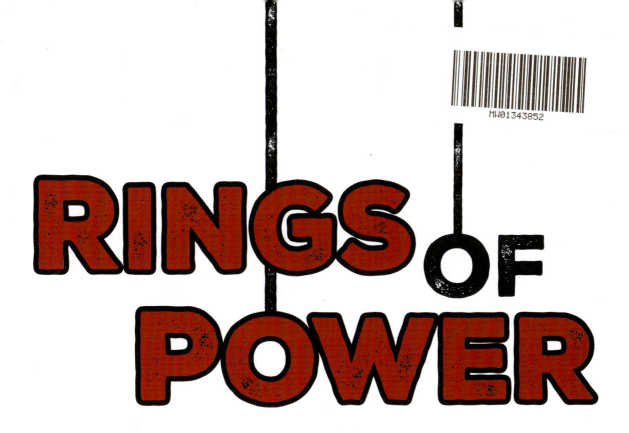

RINGS OF POWER

THE SECRETS OF SUCCESSFUL SUSPENSION TRAINING—
A SIMPLE, PROVEN SYSTEM FOR BUILDING SUSTAINABLE STRENGTH

MIKE GILLETTE

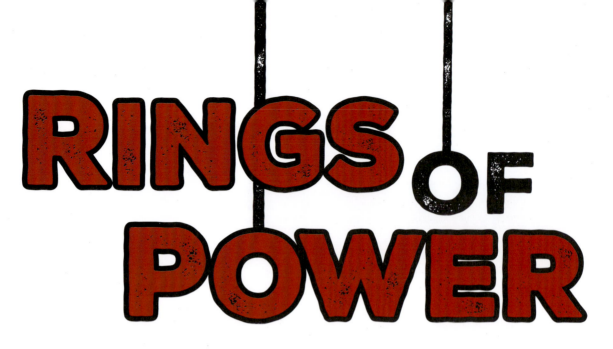

THE SECRETS OF SUCCESSFUL SUSPENSION TRAINING— A SIMPLE, PROVEN SYSTEM FOR BUILDING SUSTAINABLE STRENGTH

MIKE GILLETTE

© Copyright 2015, Mike Gillette
A Dragon Door Publications, Inc. production
All rights under International and Pan-American Copyright conventions.
Published in the United States by: Dragon Door Publications, Inc.
5 East County Rd B, #3 • Little Canada, MN 55117
Tel: (651) 487-2180 • Fax: (651) 487-3954
Credit card orders: 1-800-899-5111 • Email: support@dragondoor.com • Website: www.dragondoor.com

ISBN 10: 1942812019   ISBN 13: 978-1-942812-01-2
This edition first published in July, 2015
Printed in China

No part of this book may be reproduced in any form or by any means without the prior written consent of the Publisher, excepting brief quotes used in reviews.

Book design by Derek Brigham • www.dbrigham.com • bigd@dbrigham.com
Photography by Don Pitlik

DISCLAIMER: The authors and publisher of this material are not responsible in any manner whatsoever for any injury that may occur through following the instructions contained in this material. The activities, physical and otherwise, described herein for informational purposes only, may be too strenuous or dangerous for some people and the reader(s) should consult a physician before engaging in them. The content of this book is for informational and educational purposes only and should not be considered medical advice, diagnosis, or treatment. Readers should not disregard, or delay in obtaining, medical advice for any medical condition they may have, and should seek the assistance of their health care professionals for any such conditions because of information contained within this publication.

— Table of Contents —

Section 1 - Ring Philosophy
- Foreword 3
- Introduction 5
- The Way of the Rings 9

Section 2 - Ring Principles
- Principle 1 – Gravity 13
- Principle 2 – Ergonomics 17
- Principle 3 – Planes of Movement 19
- Principle 4 – Leverage & Loading 25
- Principle 5 – Tension as Technique 27

Section 3 - Ring Progressions
- Setting Up the Rings 31
- Horizontal Pushing 35
- Horizontal Pulling 43
- Vertical Pushing 47
- Vertical Pulling 51
- Lower-Limb Pushing 55
- Trunk Extension 59
- Trunk Flexion 63

Section 4 – Advanced Ring Concepts
- Finessing Form with the Wobble Bar 69
- Inverted Ring Progressions 81
- External Loading 85
- Ring Workouts 97

- Acknowledgments 99
- About the Author 101

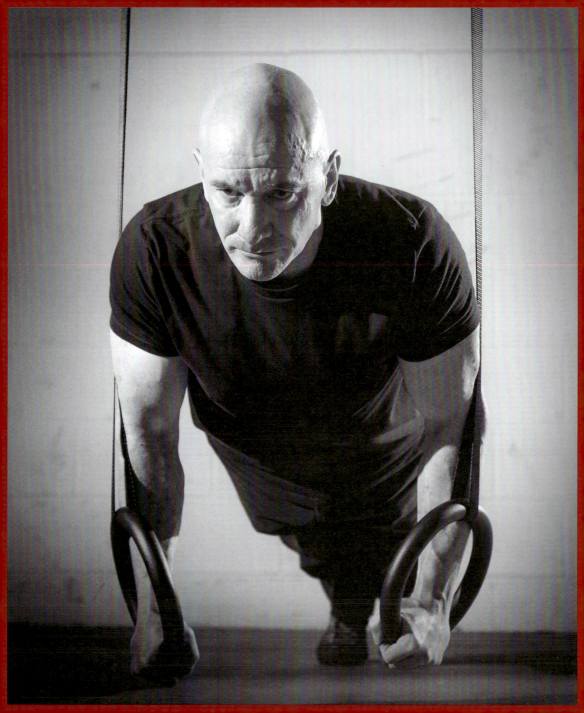

SECTION 1

RING PHILOSOPHY

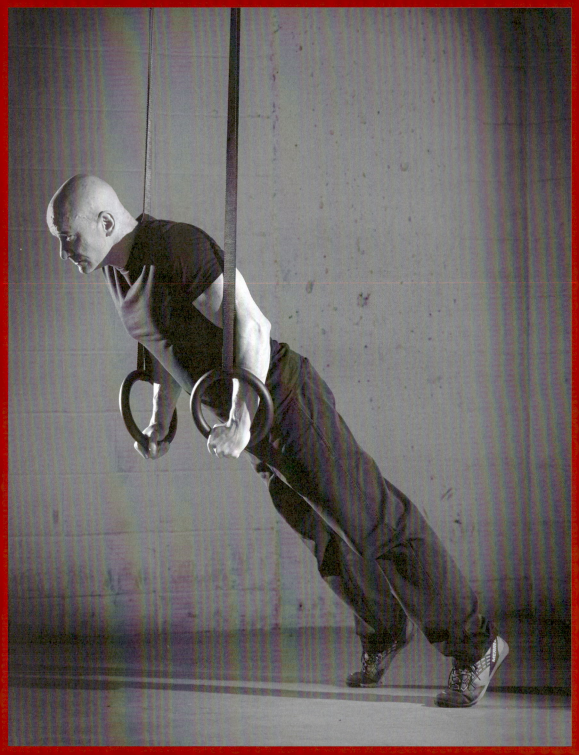

FOREWORD by DAN JOHN

I have a basic question before I decide upon buying (or stealing) a piece of equipment. It's not a long question; in fact, you should be able to memorize it easily:

Why?

Why should I buy this product? I don't want to hear that I can do this or that and this and that. I don't want to know that I can run in place with a $300 purchase as most know that running in place can be done without a lot of expense. For the kettlebell, I think it is the Swing, Goblet Squat and the TGU. For the barbell, the deadlift and the whole family of presses.

In my backyard, I have a beautiful climbing rope and a set of rings.

Why?

This book, **Rings of Power**, answers that question. Mike Gillette has made a career of learning and relearning the simple key to understanding everything in the weightroom.

And, the answer is this: Rings are a tool. Rings are a tool to build strength. Rings can fill the gap in training for areas like vertical and horizontal pulling and the need to build the abdominal wall and the Anterior Chain. Look, I love my ten-dollar ab wheel, but where do we progress from there?

Rings.

I constantly moan and complain about my athletes doing too many Bench Presses and too many Push Ups. God Bless Them for working out and a round of drinks for the whole house, but we have got to get them working in the opposite direction. How?

Rings.

Rings of Power is a strength book. **Rings of Power** focuses on some big challenges, like the Inverted Ring Push Up, but provides detailed regressions and corrections for those who might not be able to leap up on day one and pound out the repetitions.

Like me!

It's a principle-first book. Mike's point about the value of rings for most adults doing Pull Ups is spot on. For years, we have joked about MAPS, Middle Age Pull Up Syndrome. This simple, but elegant, solution can provide comfort for those who understand the need for Vertical Pulling, but can't stomach the pain of the screaming elbow. The chapter on Trunk Extension will answer all your questions concerning "what is your core?"

Many approach rings, and all pieces of gymnastics equipment, like they are only fitting for Olympic gymnasts. Mike is talking to the masses, the common man or woman who wants to be stronger and has an interest in playing with load. Your body and gravity are the load. The shaking straps will make you reconsider what you thought of as stability.

In addition to principles and the basic skills you will learn, this book is also filled with very simple-to-understand photographs. Investing in rings is very inexpensive but the payoff is amazing.

Of course, finally, I must say that a bad joke has been choking me throughout both reading the book and writing the foreword: Mike's work will indeed make you "Lord of the Rings." Thankfully, I am done with this attempt at humor.

And, a final warning: you will find yourself wanting to run and leap up on the rings. I would suggest listening to Mike and taking some baby steps up the levels of intensity and expertise. Your enthusiasm is admirable, but take your time in progression.

Enjoy. Enjoy this book and the process of relearning how to have fun while building strength.

Dan John, author, *Never Let Go*

INTRODUCTION

This is first and foremost a strength-training book. And while our training tool of choice is a piece of gymnastics equipment, this is neither a book about gymnastics or how to perform gymnastics techniques. Other than the gymnastics rings themselves, that is where any resemblance to sport gymnastics ends. The *premise* of this book is that the rings are a multi-faceted training tool. And the *purpose* of this book is to use that tool to build exceptional strength.

For many people, the whole idea of strength training is indistinct and can mean a number of different things. So before we begin talking about specific exercises or techniques, it is imperative that **you** understand just what **I** mean when the topic is **strength**.

So the first order of business is to define just what strength is and my approach for building it. After all, if we're going to be working together, we need to be on the same page and speaking the same language.

The Mike Gillette Strength Paradigm can be summed up like this… Strength starts internally and then manifests outwardly. Strong thoughts become strong goals and strong goals become strong deeds. So for you, strength should be tied into what you specifically want to accomplish. Many people will reference strength but what they're actually talking about is the visual approach to training. Meaning that they just want to look good.

Now I don't have anything negative to say about that, it just holds absolutely no interest for me as a singular goal. So when someone tells me they want to "get in shape", I will ask them what exactly they mean by that. How would you define "in shape"? Is it tied to a specific outcome? An end goal?

This sometimes has the opposite of the intended effect and leads people to look to me because they want *me* to tell *them* what their goal should be. So then I draw things out further and ask, "Okay, what do you want from *yourself*?" "What do you want out of *life*?"

Why ask such questions? Why would this have anything to do with strength? Here's why... If you want everything you can get out of life, you need to be strong. If you want long-term, healthy relationships you need to be strong for other people. If you want to achieve anything meaningful in life for yourself you need to be strong for **you**.

Here's the thing... just "looking good" doesn't get anything done in this world. Capability is what counts. So getting strong, *really* strong, can give you the ability to make yourself and your corner of the world a little bit better. How? Becoming strong makes you better. And when you're strong, you can also be strong for others. Remember that your body is *designed* to be worked hard and come back stronger. So let's begin the work of making your body fulfill its intended purpose.

Next, we need some strength-training ground rules—and this is mostly for the male readers. Women tend to grasp strength training in a purer, more mathematical way. Whereas goals for men can get blurry when bodybuilding criteria becomes confused with performance criteria. This means that men can get off course if their training is not focused on achieving their true goal.

I typically start with male <u>strength</u> clients (meaning guys who have told me that they want to focus on getting stronger) by telling them that they need to move "beyond" bodybuilding. This is because bodybuilding is the most common frame of reference for males who engage in weight training. You might be thinking, "Mike, what exactly do you mean by that?"

The answer to this is that you have to understand what bodybuilding really is. "Real" bodybuilding, (meaning competitive bodybuilding) is about many things. Sure, it's about big muscles, but it's also about having those big muscles in just the right proportions, with an accompanying low percentage of bodyfat, smooth skin, a suntan, and hopefully some charisma. So practically speaking, bodybuilding is the pursuit of an aesthetic ideal. It is a visual rather than a functional objective.

But *our* focus is the development of strength, which requires that we train outside of the bodybuilder box. That means that we say "no" to endless reps of wimpy weights, staring at ourselves in a mirror and using machines, which were solely designed to make exercises easier rather than harder.

Here is an example: Consider pull-ups. How many guys at a commercial gym do you ever see doing pull-ups? The answer is almost none. And why is that? Is it because pull-ups aren't effective? I mean, it would be easy to draw that conclusion since the typical gym has so many machines, which allow you to do all kinds of exercises *instead* of pull-ups.

The real reason most people at the gym aren't doing pull-ups is because they are **hard**. You can always find gym people lining up at the lat pull-down machine or to do some cable rows, but if you can even find a pull-up bar at your gym, I guarantee that there won't be people standing in line to use it.

But the fact remains that pull-ups are a tremendous exercise and always have been. And they're good for **everybody**... men, women, kids, everybody. So I advocate pull-ups and plenty of them. And once you have mastered pull-ups, (don't worry if you can't do a single one yet, just focus on the progressions as presented and you'll soon surprise yourself, I promise) we then find ways to make them even harder. We hang kettlebells from our waists, we strap on rucksacks full of weight plates and sometimes we even do pull-ups upside-down.

So the point here is that getting strong does not require elaborate machinery. In fact, it doesn't require *any* machines at all. Getting strong is simply about learning the right exercises, and performing them with equal parts correct technique and intensity. The 'mystery' lies in which exercises to use, and the right way to do them.

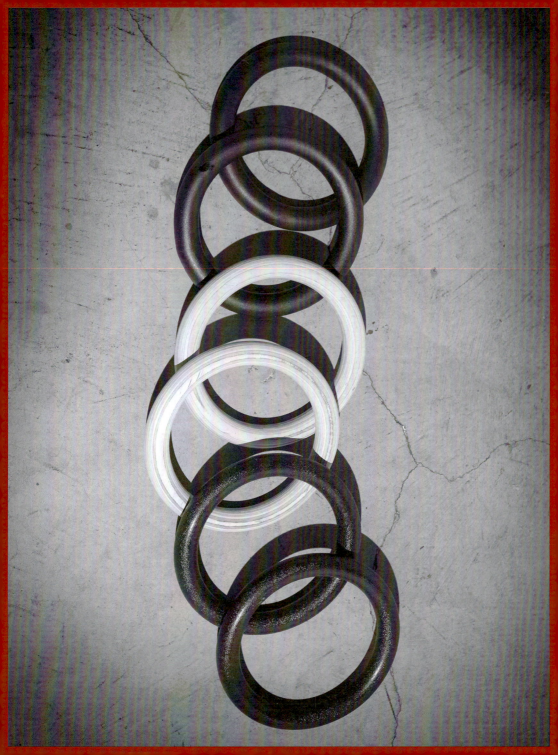

THE WAY OF THE RINGS...

The operational concept that drives my approach to the rings is what I have termed "movement-centric training". On a personal level, I had to become much more movement-focused or more accurately, *alternative* movement-focused after I turned 40. This was when I left the day-to-day world of law enforcement. I was teaching in the tactical training arena and I was also traveling more than ever before.

So my new life on the road was keeping me away from the gym much of the time. But I also had another problem, a much bigger problem. For many years I had gravitated towards certain exercises which were considered pretty standard in the gym. Things like heavy benching, pull-ups behind the head, military presses behind the head, heavy curls on the preacher bench and so on. And not only did I do those types of exercises, I did a **lot** of them. Rep after joint-grinding rep.

Now there are some guys who do all this and more and never have any injuries. Not me. After 40, my body started to make me 'pay' for focusing on what are really bodybuilding-oriented exercises. I started having problems—shoulder problems, elbow problems and wrist problems. And these new problems were wreaking havoc with my training, which combined with my travel schedule caused everything to go completely south for almost a year.

Once my work schedule calmed down and I was able to get back in the gym on a more regular basis, I *knew* I had to make some adjustments. So I stopped doing all of those things which had created so many problems for me. And believe me, that was difficult to do. After spending years developing certain habits and having once made a lot of progress with those habits... completely changing my whole way of thinking was much harder than I expected.

This led to a second very frustrating year, where I was still in a lot of pain while trying to figure out how I could maintain the strength I had developed. And more importantly, I needed to figure out how I was going to continue training productively into the future.

Little did I know that I was about to experience a physical re-birth from a couple of plastic rings and two nylon straps. In 2005 I acquired my first rings. And soon after, I was doing things with those rings which I hadn't been able to do on a conventional apparatus for several years. I was finally back to training functional movements and training them very hard without any joint pain.

The motivation I got from this was tremendous, and it led me to explore a number of other ideas using the rings. Many of those ideas are among the progressions and leverage principles which you will learn in this book.

I consider myself very fortunate to have had this second chapter in my life strength-wise. And rings were **the** pivotal step in my continued exploration of alternative methods of strength training.

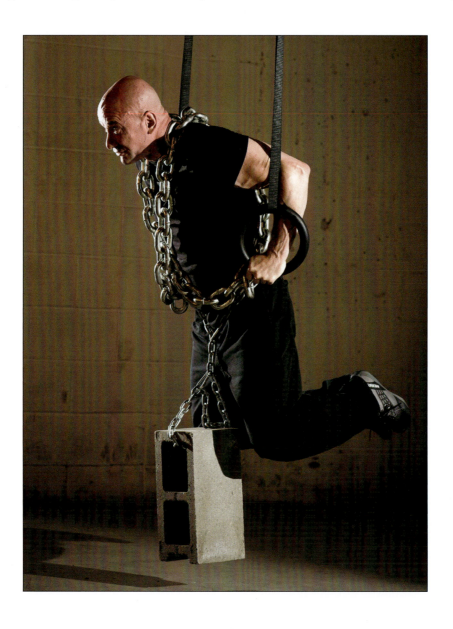

SECTION 2

RING PRINCIPLES

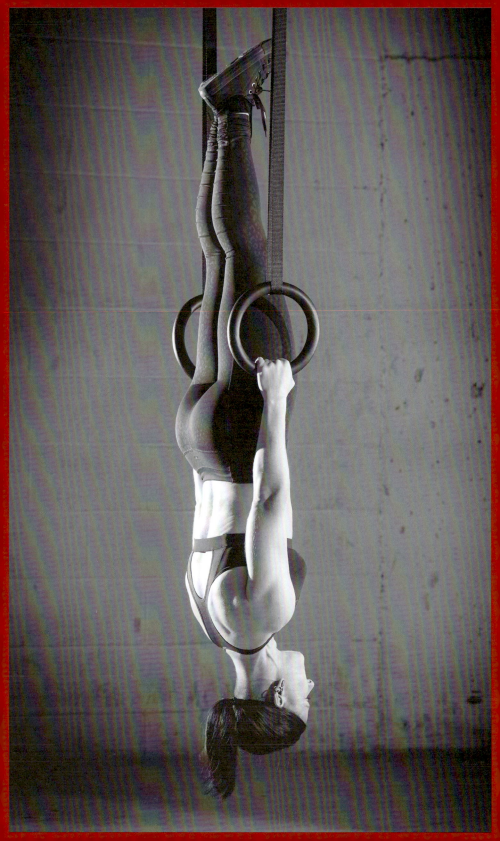

– PRINCIPLE 1 –
GRAVITY

When it comes to bodyweight or calisthenics training, exercises generally fall into two broad categories. The first category is ground-based exercises. An example of a ground-based exercise would be the humble push-up. The other category is off-the-ground exercises. Perhaps the best-known off-the-ground example would be the venerable pull-up.

In general, off-the-ground exercises tend to be harder to perform than their ground-based counterparts. This is because off-the-ground exercises almost always require supporting or moving a higher percentage of the user's total bodyweight.

Ring training falls primarily into the off-the-ground category. Exercises such as ring pull-ups or ring dips occur completely off of the ground, so this should seem logical.

But there is another critical variable to ring training that makes ring exercises fundamentally different than maneuvering one's body around a fixed, horizontal bar. And that variable is oscillation.

Oscillation can be best understood as a pendulum-like, swinging motion. And this motion occurs in response to too much movement on the part of a person attempting to perform a given ring exercise.

The only cure for excessive oscillation is stronger, more precise movements. In other words, getting stronger will require practice. And with practice comes not only more strength but also more *control*. Ring training enhances overall athleticism by not only making your movement stronger, but also by making your movement ***better***.

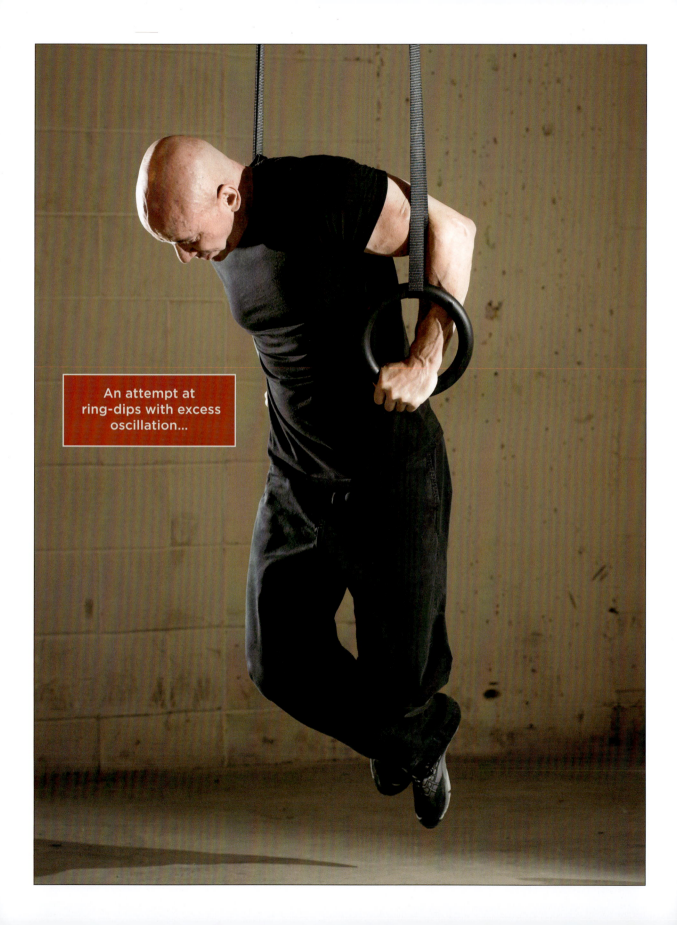

An attempt at ring-dips with excess oscillation...

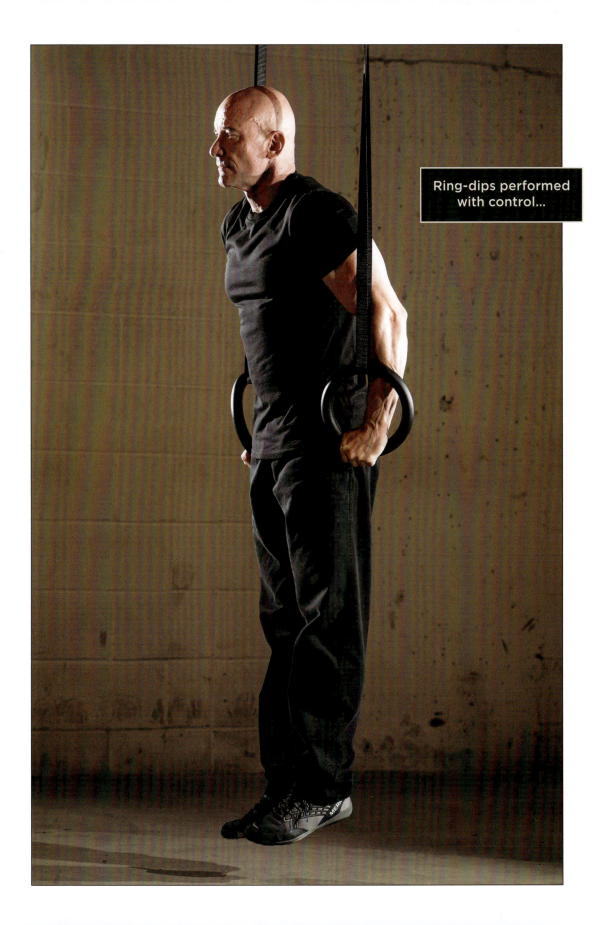

Ring-dips performed with control...

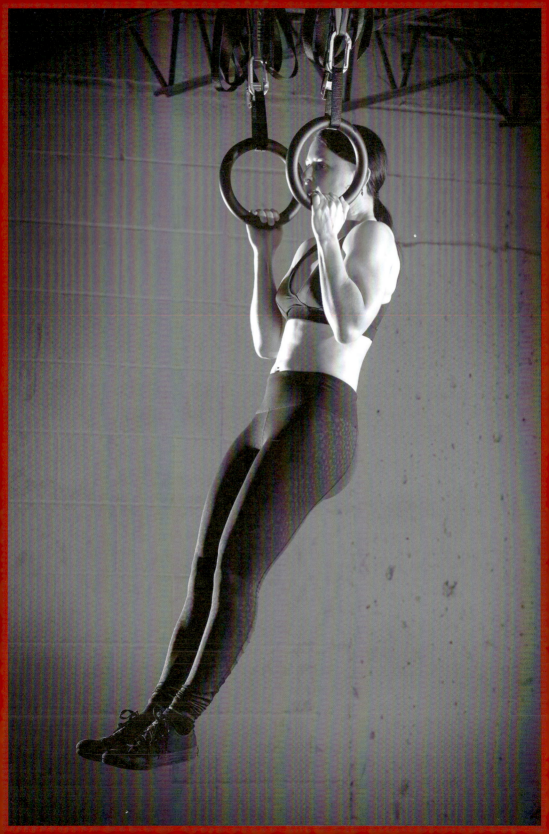

– PRINCIPLE 2 –
ERGONOMICS

rgonomics is the study of functional design. Specifically, the design of things that people physically interact with. When an item has been designed in a way that makes it more efficient or safe to operate, then it is described as ergonomic.

I describe ring training as an ergonomic activity performed with ergonomic tools. It is precisely the user-friendly characteristics of ring training which led me back to the serious pursuit of strength.

Ring training is ergonomic in nature because the apparatus adjusts to the individual in a way that is not seen with any barbell, pull-up bar or allegedly-adjustable exercise machine. Earlier, when I recounted my difficulty with straight bar pull-ups, it was the bar itself that caused me problems. The long immovable bar does not allow my wrists or elbows to move and the result is that I experience considerable pain in those joints if I attempt to perform pull-ups on a bar.

However, when I perform a pull-up on the rings, my arms rotate to a neutral position. No stress is transferred to the joints and everything from my wrists to my shoulders feel great. And no matter if I'm doing ring push-ups, ring-dips or handstand push-ups on the rings, I experience no joint problems whatsoever.

This is significant, because if I recreate those same motions using a barbell or parallel bars in the case of dips, I experience almost immediate pain in those joints. Rings put the stress where you want it—on the working muscles.

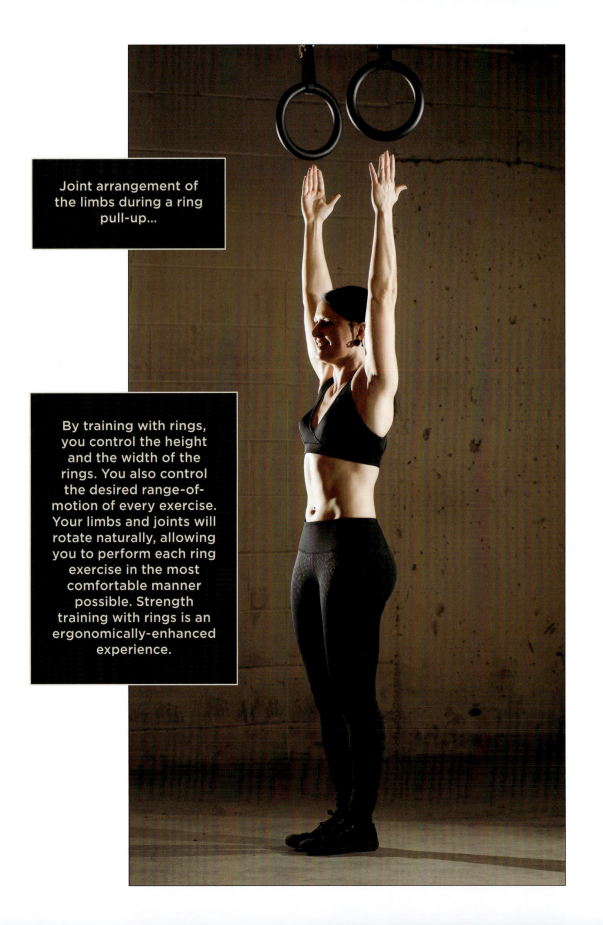

Joint arrangement of the limbs during a ring pull-up...

By training with rings, you control the height and the width of the rings. You also control the desired range-of-motion of every exercise. Your limbs and joints will rotate naturally, allowing you to perform each ring exercise in the most comfortable manner possible. Strength training with rings is an ergonomically-enhanced experience.

– PRINCIPLE 3 –
PLANES OF MOVEMENT

lanes of movement constitute the building blocks of ring strength development. In very basic terms we are talking about understanding how the body moves and the optimal way to use rings to train yourself to move powerfully.

At a basic level, the body performs several common movement tasks. Of course there are infinite subtle variations, but the following seven movement planes encompass the broad spectrum of movement potential.

With the upper body... there is vertical pushing, vertical pulling, horizontal pushing and horizontal pulling.

With the lower body... there is lower-limb pushing, posterior chain movements and anterior chain movements. So let's break these down with an exercise example of each.

PRIMARY MOVEMENT PATTERNS

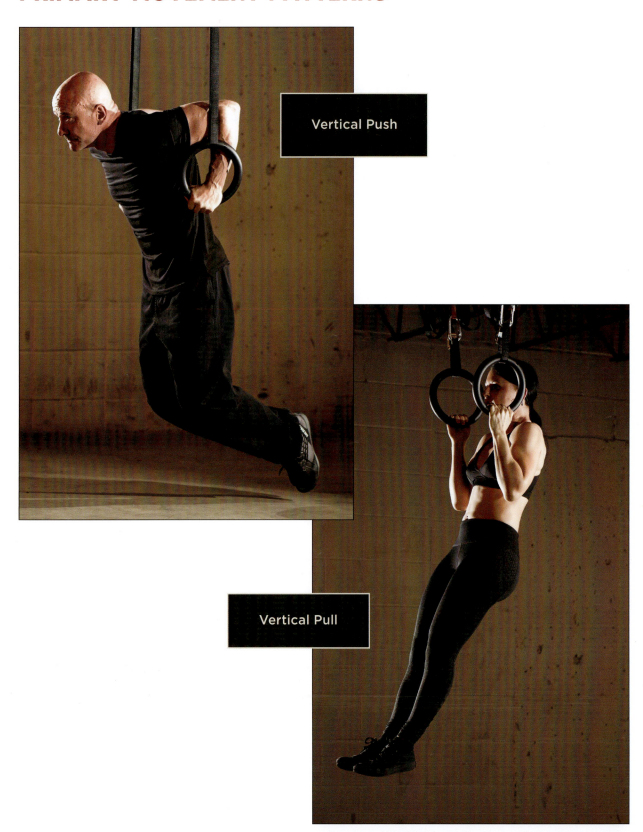

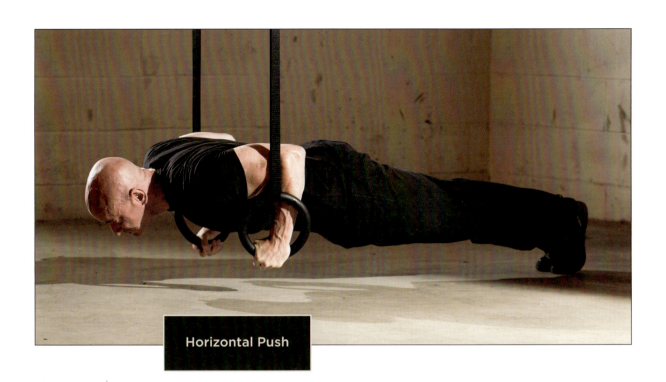

Horizontal Push

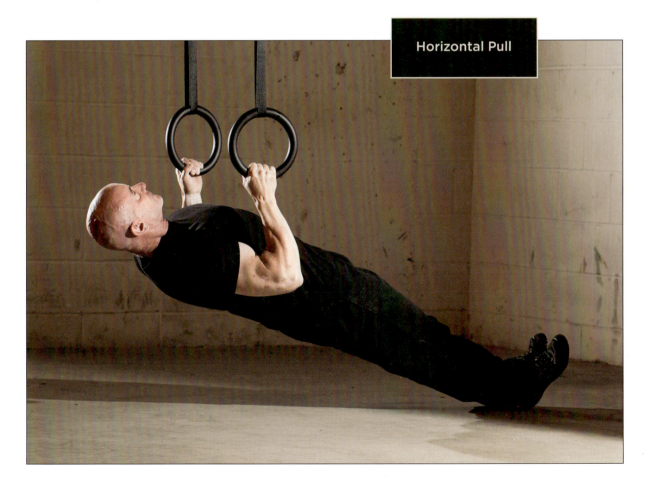

Horizontal Pull

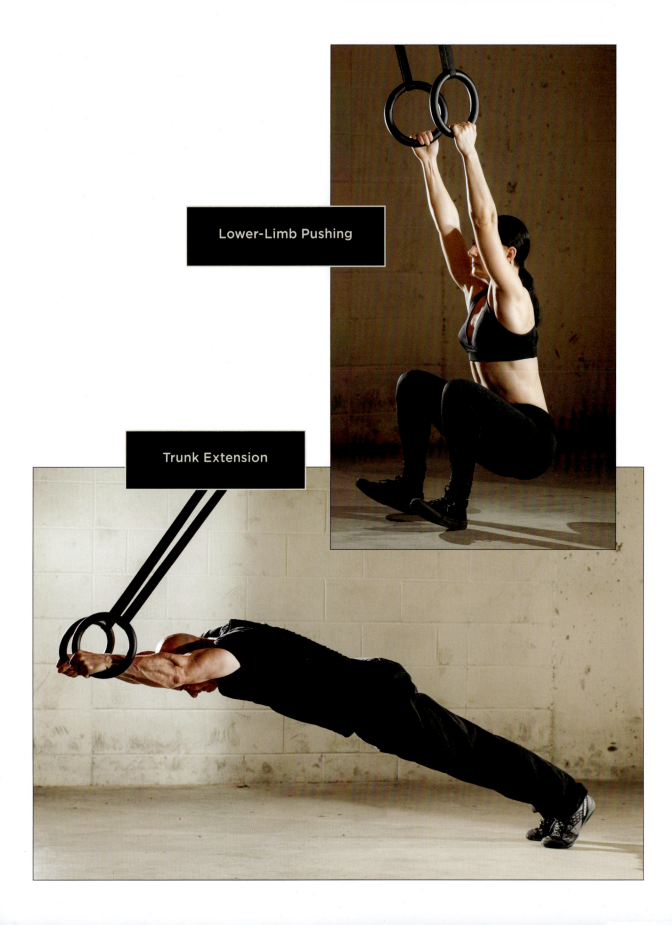

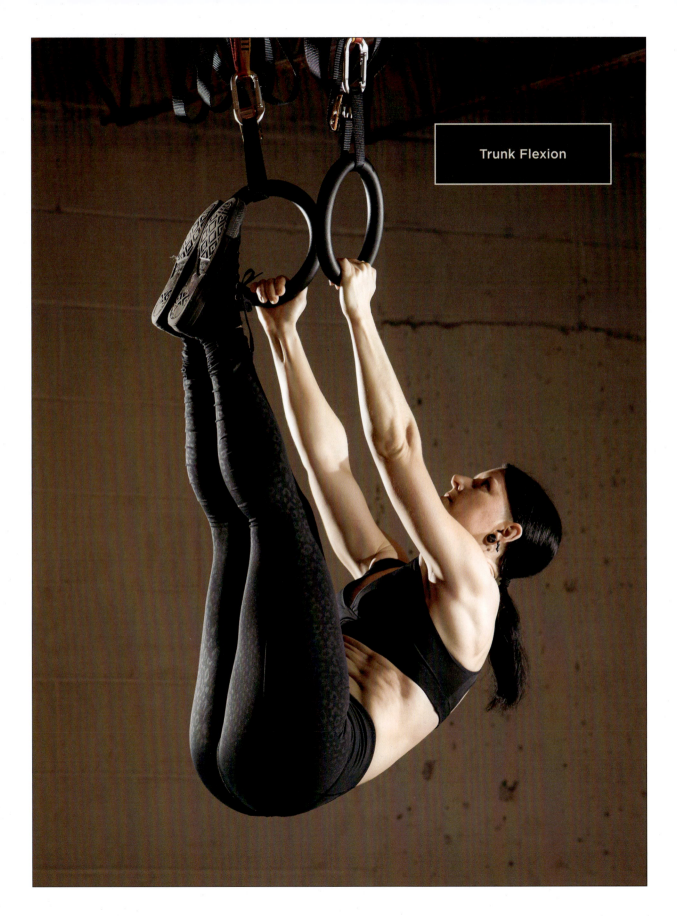
Trunk Flexion

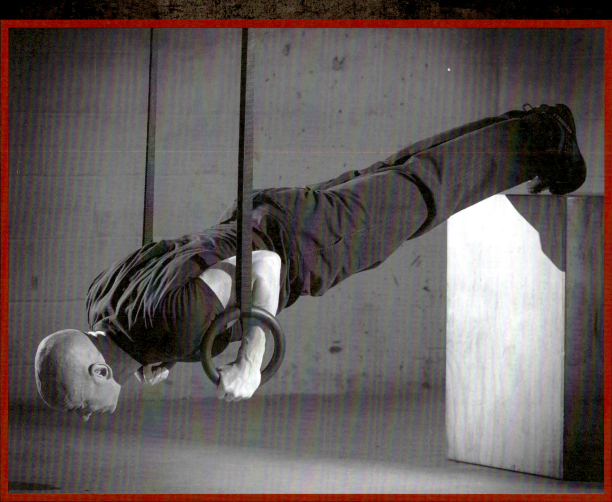

– PRINCIPLE 4 –
LEVERAGE & LOADING

Ring training, like weightlifting, is a form of resistance training. For the most part, the resistance is provided by the user's own bodyweight. But what makes ring training such a sophisticated approach to strength-building is how infinitely adjustable that resistance can be.

Part of this adjustability is inherent in the design of the rings themselves. By making slight adjustments up and down the webbing, it is a simple matter to alter the intensity of a given exercise. These "intensity alterations" involve understanding how the principle of leverage applies to ring training.

In ring training, leverage manipulation is how we control **loading**. First, we need to understand conventional loading as applied to resistance training. We refer to this as 'actual load'. An example of actual load is placing two 100-pound weight plates onto a 45-pound barbell. The actual load of that barbell if you were to lift it off of the ground is 245 *actual* pounds.

Leverage manipulation works differently. Manipulating leverage relates to a concept I refer to as *"perceived load"*. Perceived load relates to how difficult an exercise is based on the way you adjust the relationships of the angles involved. Based on these angle adjustments, the exercise and its accompanying load feels heavier or lighter. Here is an example...

Performing strongmen often do something called leverage lifting. They will pick up a sledgehammer by grasping the very bottom of the handle. Then they will extend the hammer upwards, forwards, or even behind them. This is a very difficult feat because a standard 16-pound sledgehammer feels heavier and heavier as you move your grip down the handle and away from the weighted sledge portion.

The most extreme examples of this are the legendary leverage feats attributed to a strongman named Slim "The Hammerman" Farman. Slim performed feats with a custom-built pair of sledgehammers. These hammers had *extra* weight plates attached to the heads and handles which were 31" long.

Slim would pick these hammers up at the very end of the handles. Then he would extend his arms completely straight forward and locked out. He would then allow the sledgehammers to slowly tip down towards his face and touch his nose while his arms remained locked. Any break in concentration or a momentary muscular failure would have split his skull and snapped his wrists like twigs.

Here's the key point—Slim grabbed these hammers by the very end of the handles and held them at arm's length which created an unbelievable 1,736 pounds of pressure on his wrists.

I will pause here for a moment so that you may digest just how incredible this feat is. The take-away is that exercise loading via leverage-manipulation has real-world application to strength training. It is also the primary variable we will use to help deconditioned beginners get on the road to impressive strength.

Leverage manipulation can be utilized to make an exercise like this push-up variation easier to perform.

Alternatively, leverage manipulation can be used to make an exercise more challenging, as shown in this push-up variation.

– PRINCIPLE 5 –
TENSION AS TECHNIQUE

One of the most beneficial aspects of ring training is the unique way that it literally "teaches" you to attain correct body mechanics and postural integrity. Now, this is not to say that you can't deliberately perform ring exercises incorrectly. You certainly can. But there is a performance paradox at work here—it is actually more difficult to perform these exercises the wrong way than the right way.

You can try an example of what I'm talking about right now on the floor. Put yourself in the starting position of a push-up. Concentrate on tightening up your body from your toes to your shoulders. Make a concerted effort to tighten up the muscles of your feet, calves, hamstrings, glutes, abdomen, and all the way up the back. Now, with your body "pre-loaded" with muscular tension, perform a push-up. Assuming that you are already strong enough to execute at least a few push-ups, you should find that this "muscles-tensed" process allows you to pop up and down with a marked efficiency-of-effort.

Now, to experience the "wrong" way to exercise, try another push-up or a few. But this time don't focus on being tight. Rather, try to push yourself up while maintaining a "slack" middle and without tension in the legs or midsection. Most people find that in addition to a very poor-looking push-up, it takes more effort to push the body upwards in this manner. By eliminating the tension you created a moment earlier, you have turned your body into what could be described as "dead weight". It is the same phenomena as lifting a duffle bag full of sand. The weight is hard to manage due to the "shapeless" nature of the container.

Ring training takes this tension phenomena and essentially magnifies it. It's one thing to have a slack body while resting on the floor but it's an entirely different thing to experience while supporting yourself above that same floor on a set of rings.

There is an adage in the world of gymnastics that sums up this concept very succinctly, "Tight is light". The key performance variable of all the ring strength exercises is intentional control of muscular tension. So, you know you're doing an exercise "right" when you've learned how to keep your body **tight**.

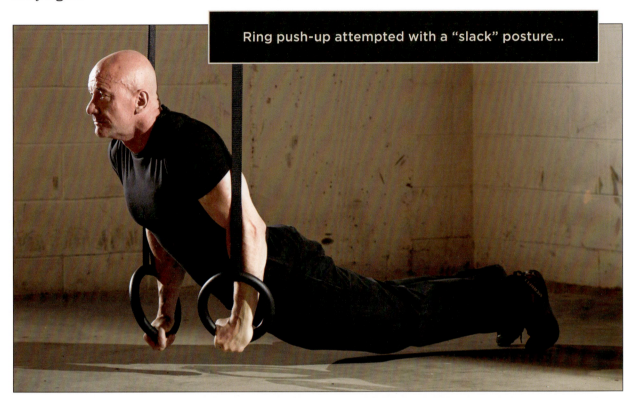

Ring push-up attempted with a "slack" posture...

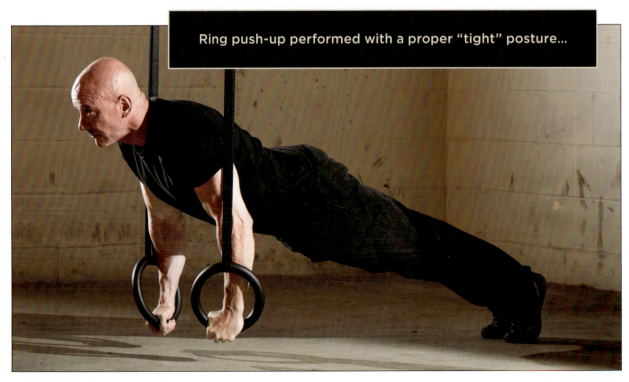

Ring push-up performed with a proper "tight" posture...

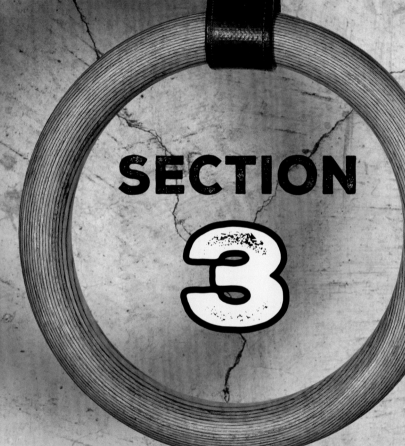

SECTION 3

RING PROGRESSIONS

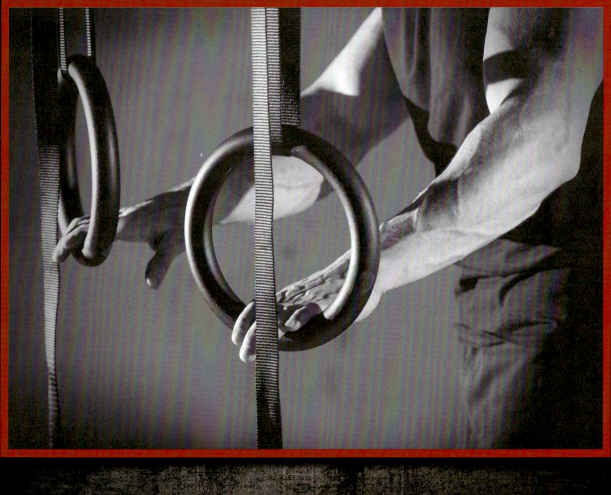

SETTING UP THE RINGS

The importance of knowing how to set up your rings correctly cannot be overstated. Your safety as well as that of your clients depends on it.

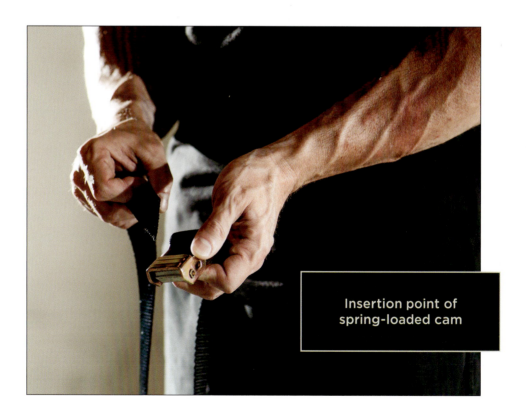

Insertion point of spring-loaded cam

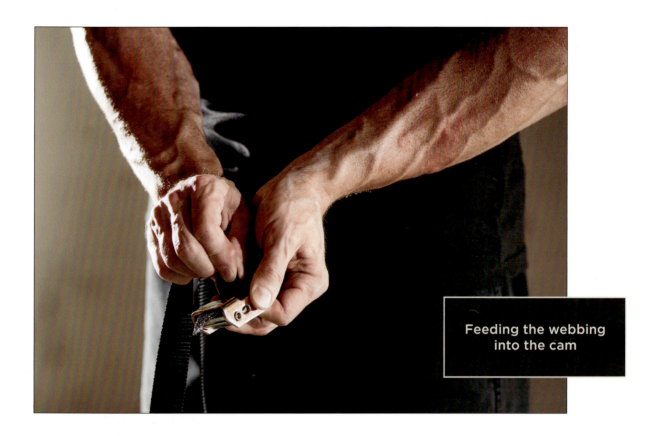

Feeding the webbing into the cam

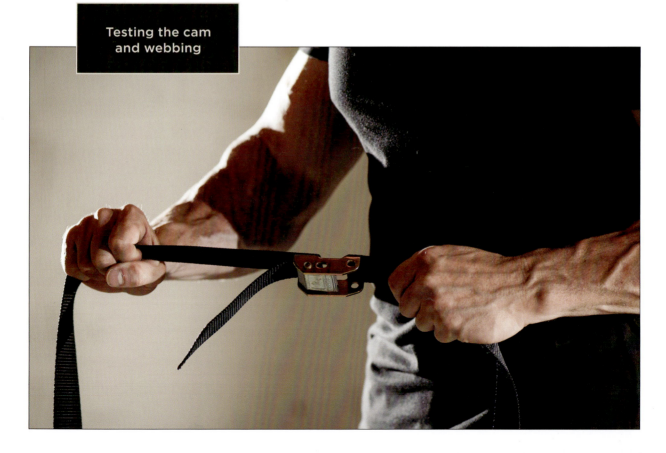

Testing the cam and webbing

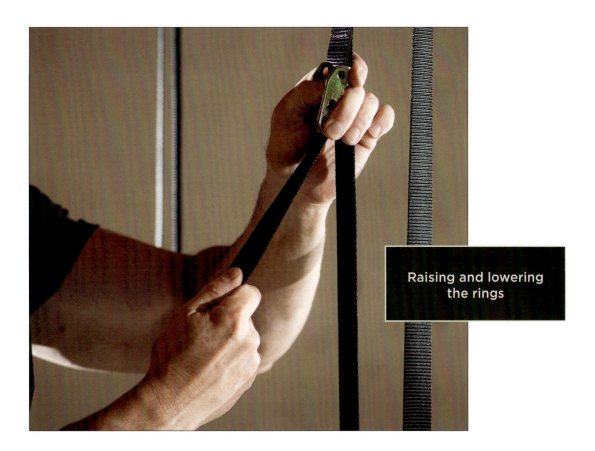

Raising and lowering the rings

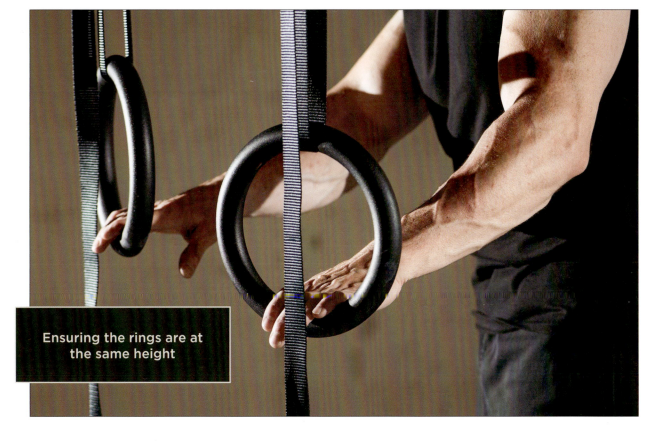

Ensuring the rings are at the same height

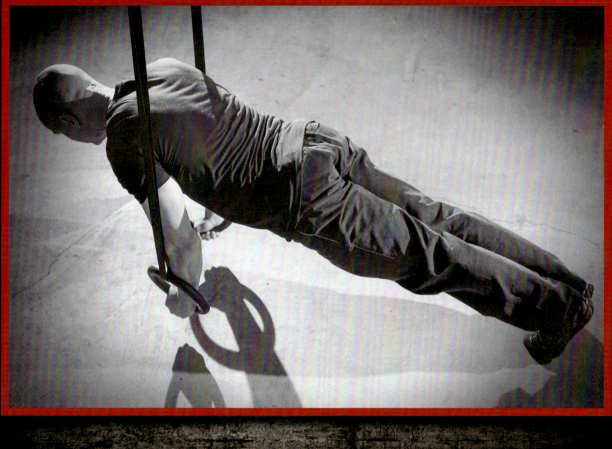

HORIZONTAL PUSHING
– THE RING PUSH-UP –

This first progression will probably seem the most familiar to you. We will be recreating the posture and movements of the push-up, except that we'll be doing it on the rings. Unlike a conventional push-up, we can use the rings to control the exercise's range-of-motion to a far greater degree.

SET-UP

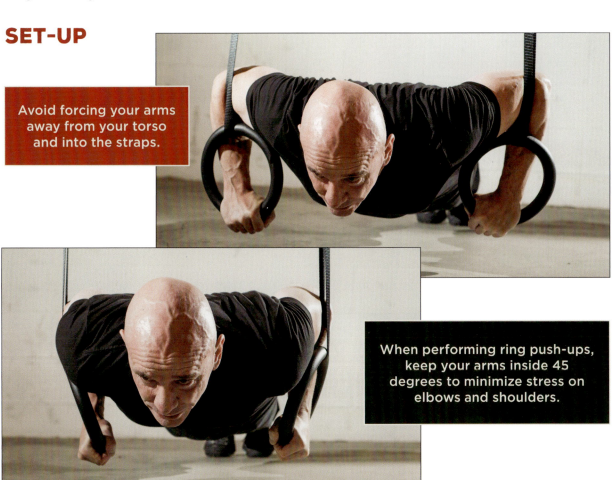

Avoid forcing your arms away from your torso and into the straps.

When performing ring push-ups, keep your arms inside 45 degrees to minimize stress on elbows and shoulders.

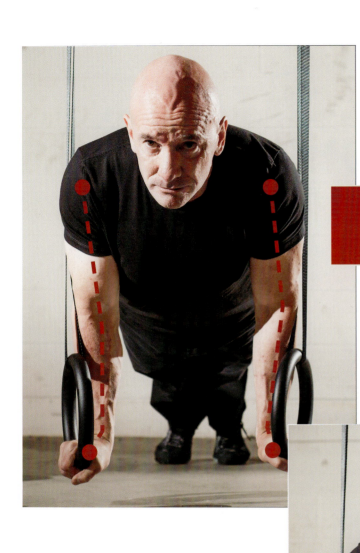

Don't let the wrists bend.

When performing ring push-ups, keep your hands, wrists and forearms aligned...

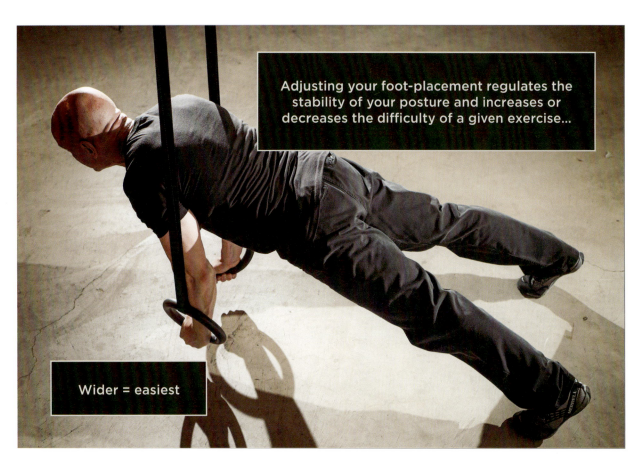

Adjusting your foot-placement regulates the stability of your posture and increases or decreases the difficulty of a given exercise...

Wider = easiest

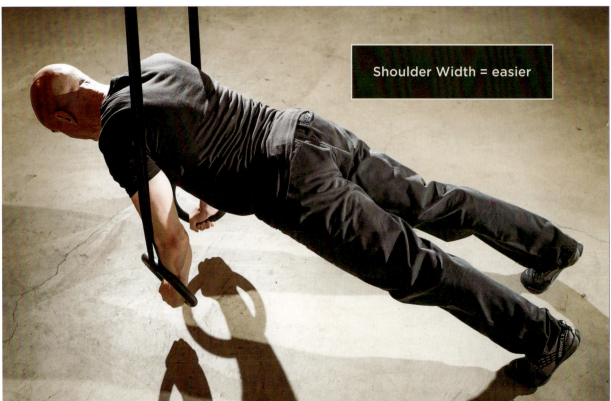

Shoulder Width = easier

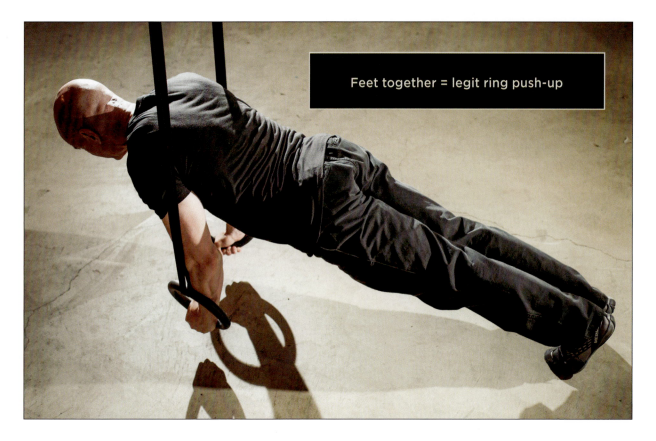

Feet together = legit ring push-up

FINDING YOUR STARTING POINT...

Now that you know how to set up your equipment for safety, it's time to learn how to set yourself up for success with the safe and successful execution of a ring push-up. Within each progression you will be shown three exercise variations. Each variation represents a different level of difficulty. The final variation will be the "standard" version of a given exercise.

Note that you are never limited to just the three examples of each variation shown in this book. These three variations merely demonstrate the almost limitless nature of ring training. The only "limit" is the space available in this book to demonstrate all of the possibilities.

Some of you may need to adjust an exercise or two to an even easier version than the "easy" version in the book. If this is you, don't be discouraged. The point is to start at your current level and progress from there.

So let's get started...

RING PUSH-UP: VARIATION #1

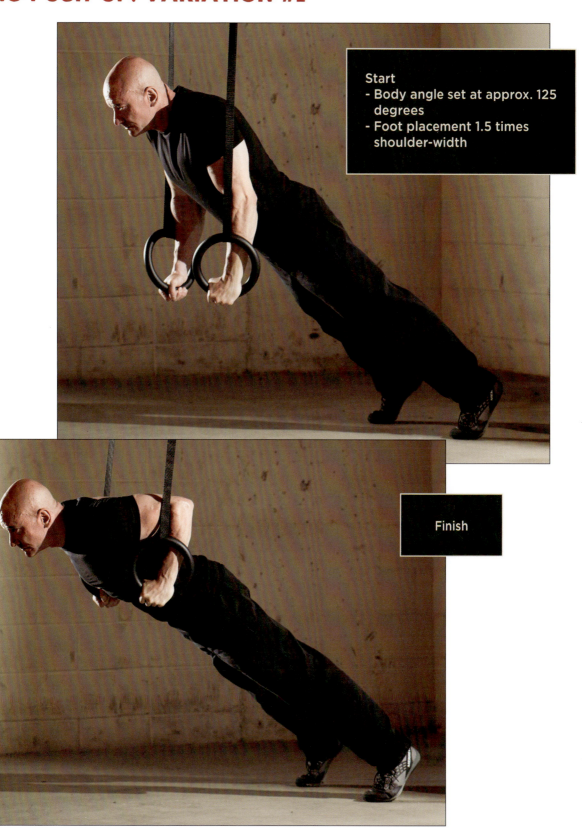

Start
- Body angle set at approx. 125 degrees
- Foot placement 1.5 times shoulder-width

Finish

RING PUSH-UP: VARIATION #2

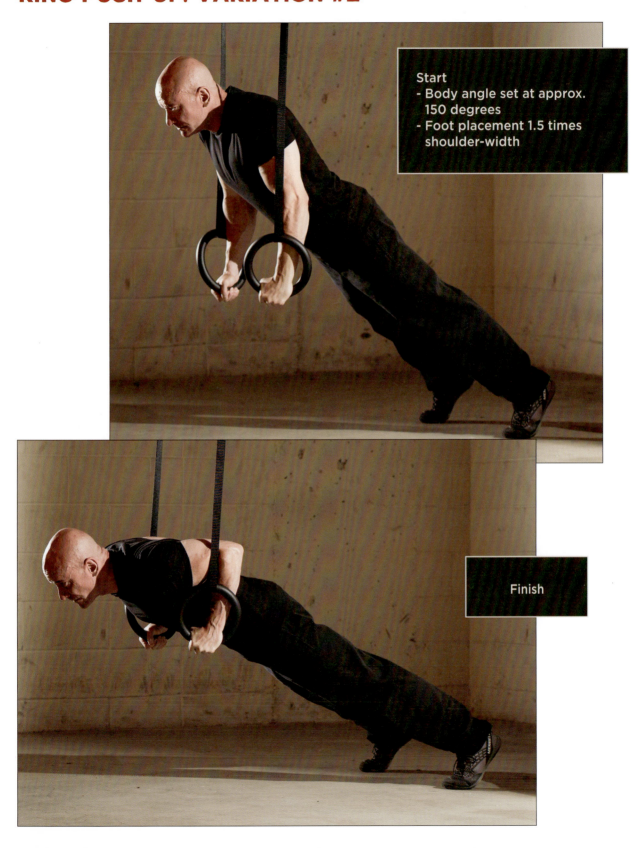

Start
- Body angle set at approx. 150 degrees
- Foot placement 1.5 times shoulder-width

Finish

RING PUSH-UP: VARIATION #3

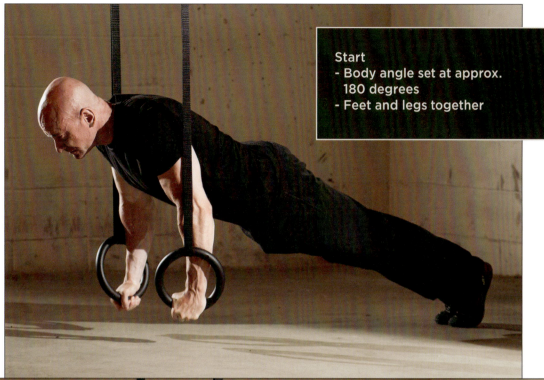

Start
- Body angle set at approx. 180 degrees
- Feet and legs together

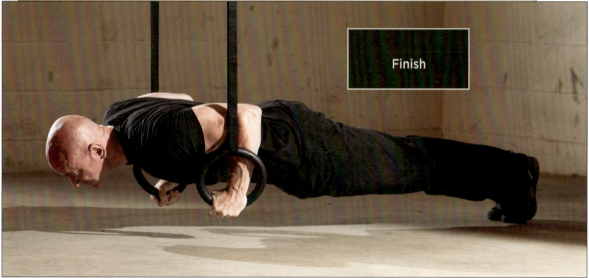

Finish

RING PUSH-UP POINTS-OF-PERFORMANCE:

- Maintain a straight body line from heels to shoulders
- Don't hyperextend the neck
- Keep tight
- If reps are sloppy, re-set the rings to a height that allows clean reps

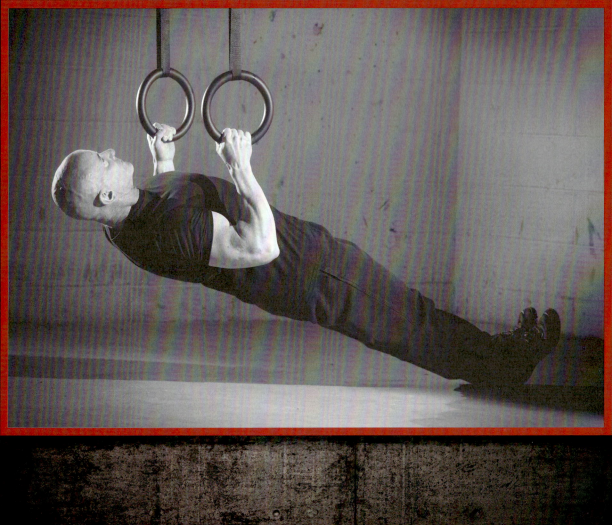

HORIZONTAL PULLING
– THE RING ROW –

SET-UP

Start by spacing the rings shoulder-width apart. Set the rings at a height which will challenge you, but still allows you to perform six to ten quality repetitions. In the beginning stages this may require some experimentation as you dial in your optimum starting position.

Grasp the rings with your palms facing each other. Then walk yourself forward or back until you are at the desired angle to begin the movement. Rest your weight on your heels, toes pointed up. Your heels will serve as the fulcrum point of the exercise. Assume the starting position with your arms straight and maintain a straight body line as you raise and lower yourself.

RING ROW: VARIATION #1

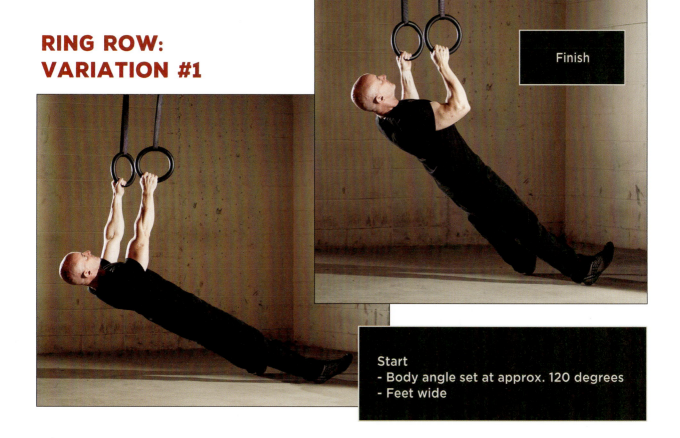

Finish

Start
- Body angle set at approx. 120 degrees
- Feet wide

RING ROW: VARIATION #2

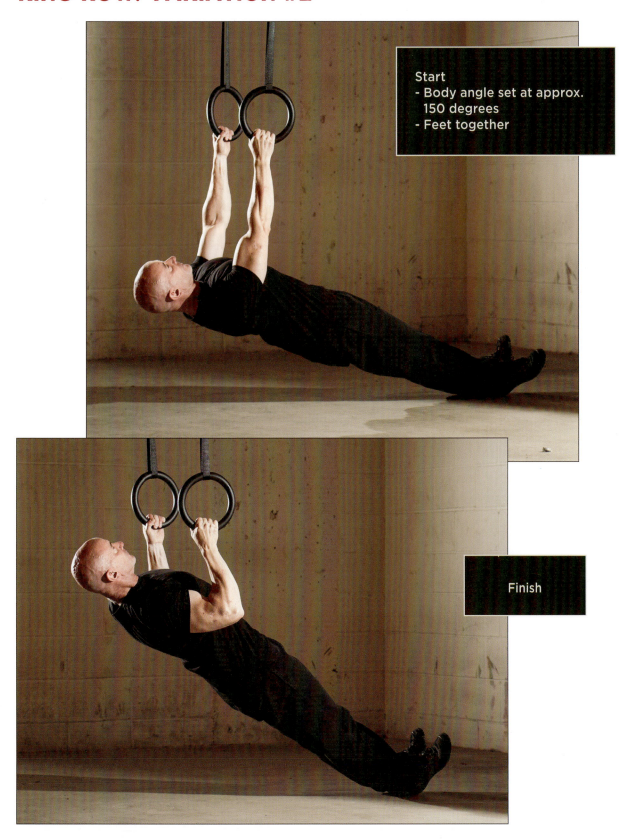

Start
- Body angle set at approx. 150 degrees
- Feet together

Finish

RING ROW: VARIATION #3

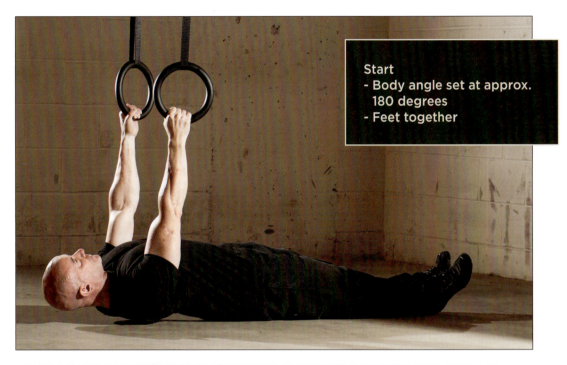

Start
- Body angle set at approx. 180 degrees
- Feet together

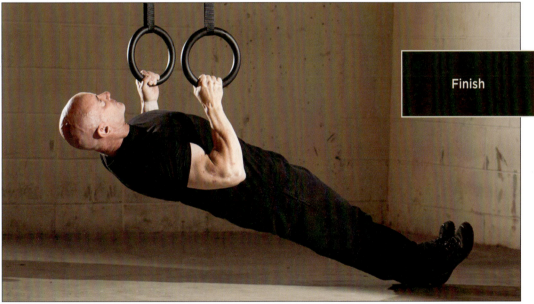

Finish

RING ROW POINTS-OF-PERFORMANCE:

- Maintain a straight body line from heels to shoulders
- Pull yourself up by drawing the elbows back and contracting the back muscles rather than just emphasizing the arms
- Keep tight
- If reps are sloppy, check yourself and re-set the rings

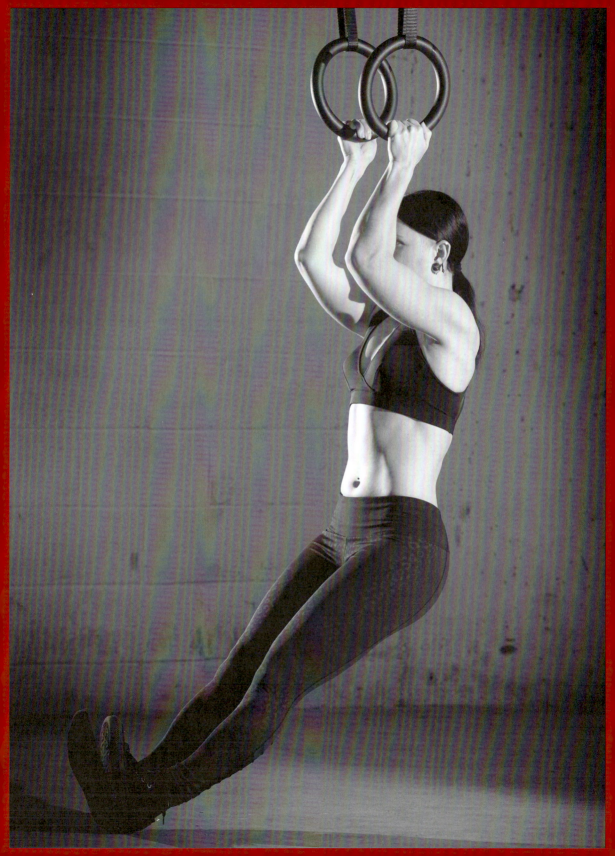

VERTICAL PULLING
– THE RING PULL-UP –

SET-UP

Set-up is a pivotal part of ring pull-up performance. If you are not ready to perform an unassisted ring pull-up yet, you will need to obtain a sturdy object for support. This will be something you can rest your feet on in order to adjust the "load" of the exercise. A weight bench, plyo box or a sturdy chair will work. Remember that a wider object will provide more options for foot placement. The ultimate considerations for whatever item you choose is the durability and stability of that item. Safety first...

When grasping the rings, take ahold of them as though you are grabbing a horizontal bar with an overhand grip. As you pull yourself up, your wrists and elbows will rotate to some degree. It is typical to find your palms facing each other at the top of the repetition. There is no "wrong" hand position with this exercise, they will simply move with the rings between the start and finish positions.

RING PULL-UP: VARIATION #1

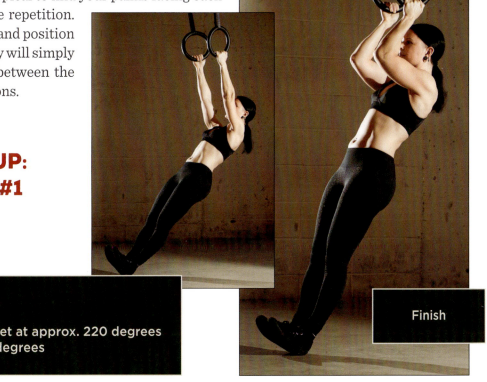

Start
- Body angle set at approx. 220 degrees
- Trunk at 90 degrees

Finish

RING PULL-UP: VARIATION #2

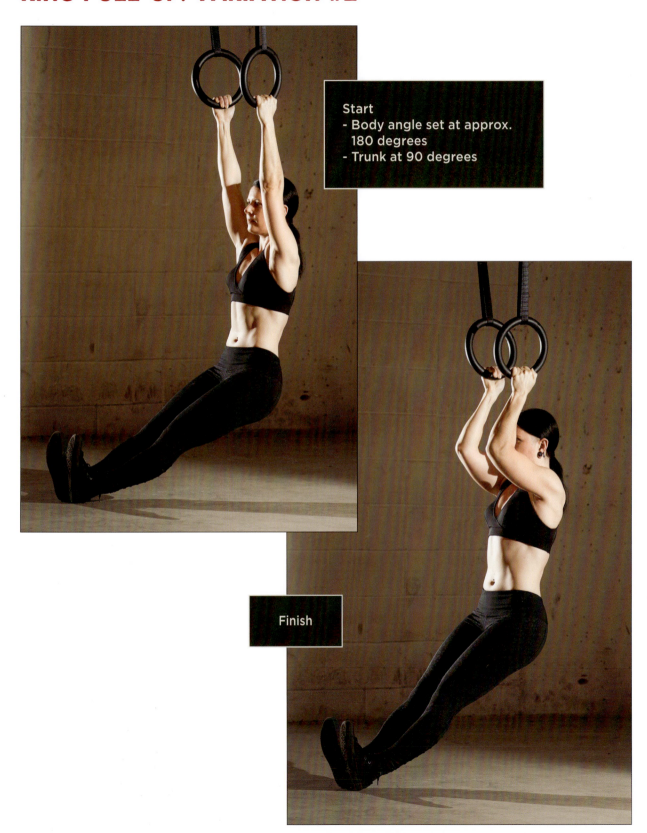

Start
- Body angle set at approx. 180 degrees
- Trunk at 90 degrees

Finish

RING PULL-UP: VARIATION #3

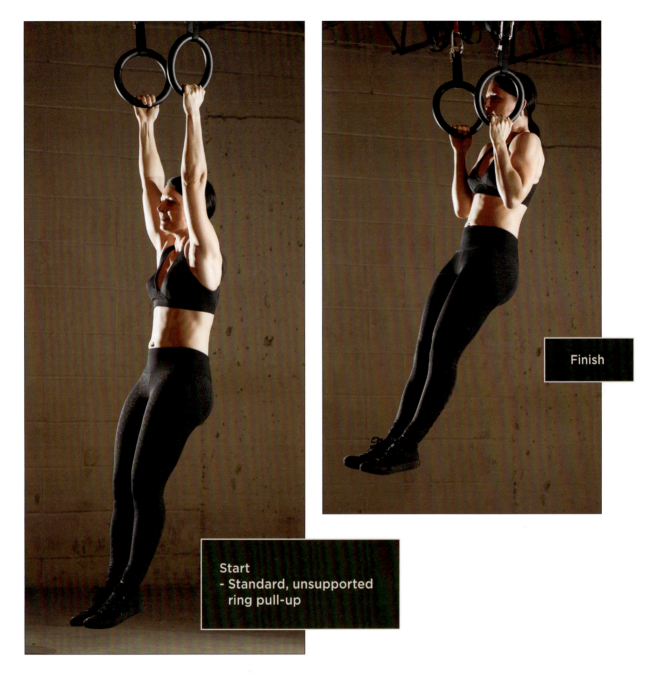

Start
- Standard, unsupported ring pull-up

Finish

RING PULL-UP POINTS-OF-PERFORMANCE:

- Keep the trunk oriented vertically, even during the supported variations
- Avoid arching the back, maintain a neutral spine
- Don't tilt the head back or "reach upwards" with the chin
- Keep tight (always!)
- If reps fall short of the rings, return to a variation that you can perform with proper form

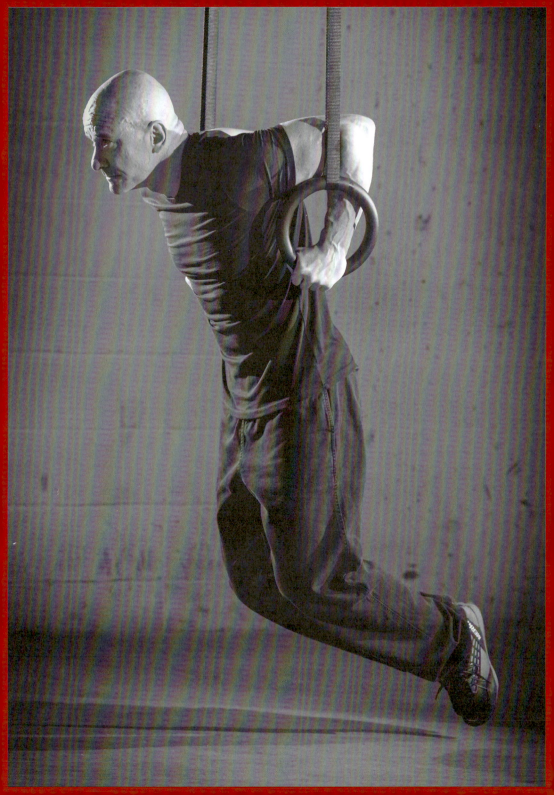

VERTICAL PUSHING
– THE RING DIP –

SET-UP

If you utilized some type of support for ring pull-ups, then you may want to use the same support for the ring-dip progression.

Start by positioning yourself directly under and inside the rings. Grasp the rings firmly and make sure that you keep the bones of the forearm aligned with the wrist. People with weaker wrists have a tendency to let their wrists "drop" which results in the fists pushing out, perpendicular to the body. Avoid dropping the wrists inward as it leads to immediate discomfort and long-term injury.

While performing the supported ring-dip variations, ensure that the trunk is upright and that you maintain a neutral spine. Keep your hands aligned with the hips as you begin the descending phase. Leaning forward excessively can stress the shoulders, so keep this visual/tactile point of reference to maintain quality-control of your repetitions. At the "bottom" of the ring-dip, ensure that your upper arms are parallel with the floor. Descending beyond this point can be stressful to the elbow joints.

RING DIP: VARIATION #1

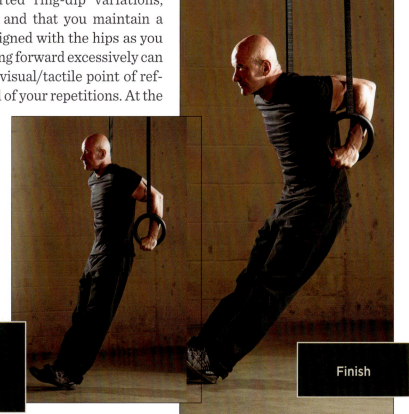

Start
- Legs at approx. 220 degrees
- Feet supported

Finish

RING DIP: VARIATION #2

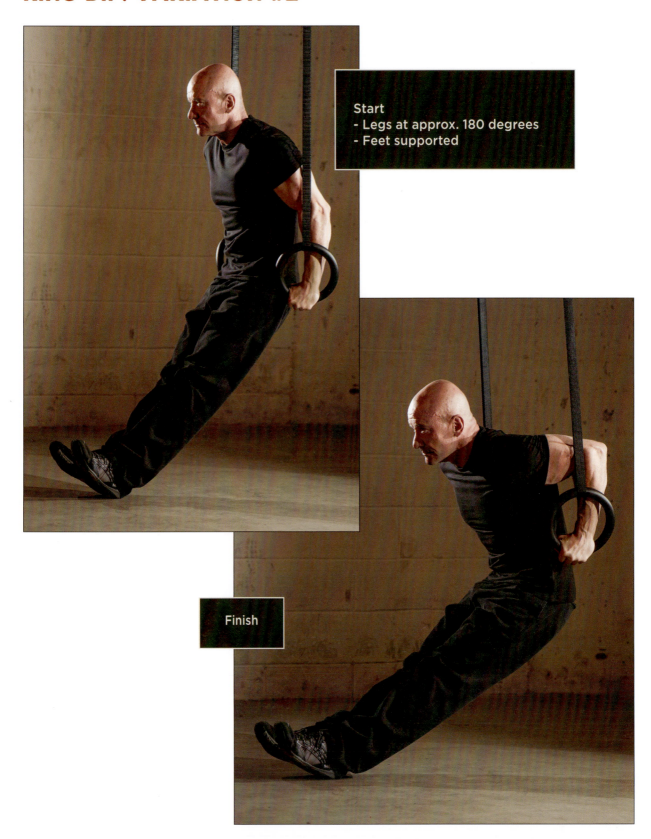

Start
- Legs at approx. 180 degrees
- Feet supported

Finish

RING DIP: VARIATION #3

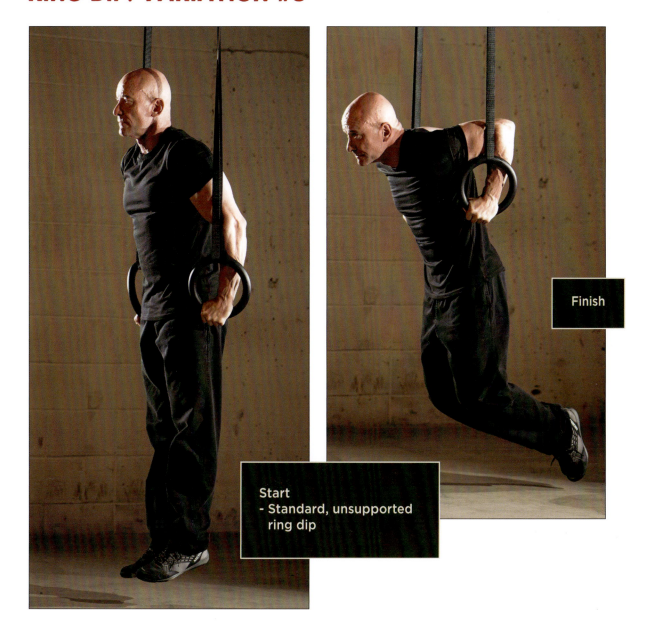

Start
- Standard, unsupported ring dip

Finish

RING DIP POINTS-OF-PERFORMANCE:

- Keep the trunk oriented vertically, even during the supported variations
- Avoid arching the back, maintain a neutral spine
- Don't tilt forwards beyond 90 degrees
- Keep elbows tight to the body
- Don't descend past 180 degrees
- Train at your your current level. If the reps aren't clean, fall back to a variation you can perform with good technique.

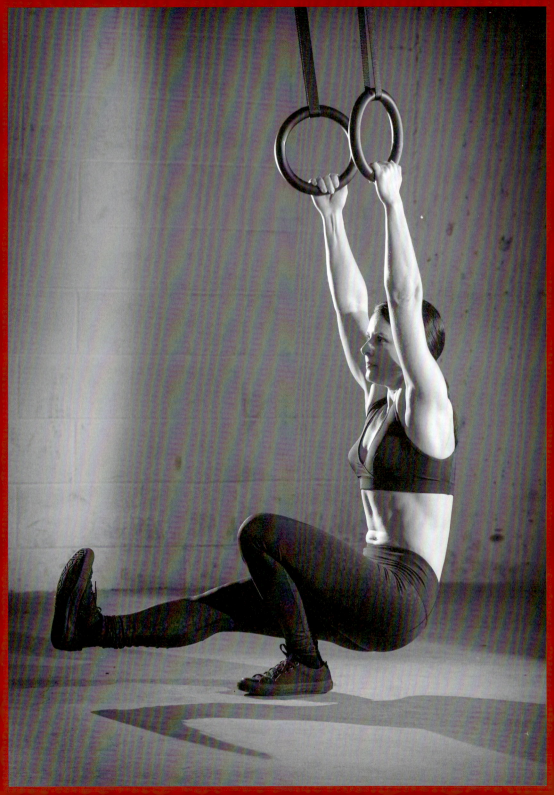

LOWER-LIMB PUSHING
– THE RING SQUAT –

SET-UP

When it comes to lower-limb training, the rings play more of a supporting role. Key to setting up the rings for the ring squat series is making sure that the support structure for your rings is both vertically and horizontally stable. This is necessary because most of the force on the rings during this progression is exerted laterally. If you are using a freestanding pull-up bar for your other ring progressions, test it for stability before attempting this exercise series.

To start, position the rings at an angle to the overhead support. You will need enough slack in the webbing to allow an angle of approximately 150 degrees. Grasp the rings while keeping the arms straight. Your arms will be supporting you as you lean against the rings. The arms should stay relaxed to help you find your ideal balance point as well as reduce unnecessary fatigue in the arms. As you lean back into your preferred starting position, put your weight back into your heels. Try to raise your toes slightly upwards and imagine driving your heels into the floor on each rep.

One of the anatomical benefits of ring squats is that they minimize stress on the knee joint as compared to conventional squats. The rings allow you to position yourself so that your shins are oriented vertically. Although this makes ring squats more comfortable for the knee *joints*, the leg *muscles* will not be nearly so lucky.

RING SQUAT: VARIATION #1

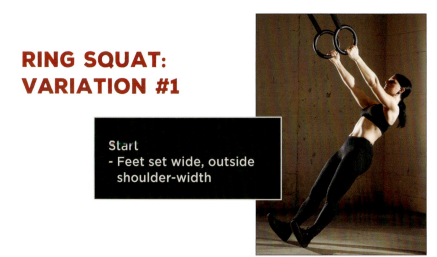

Start
- Feet set wide, outside shoulder-width

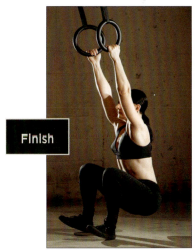

Finish

RING SQUAT: VARIATION #2

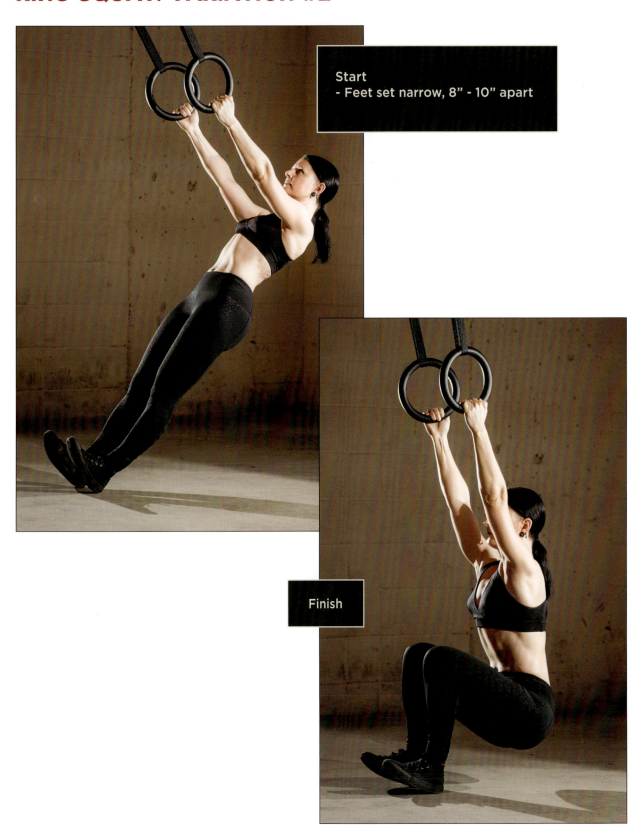

Start
- Feet set narrow, 8" - 10" apart

Finish

RING SQUAT: VARIATION #3

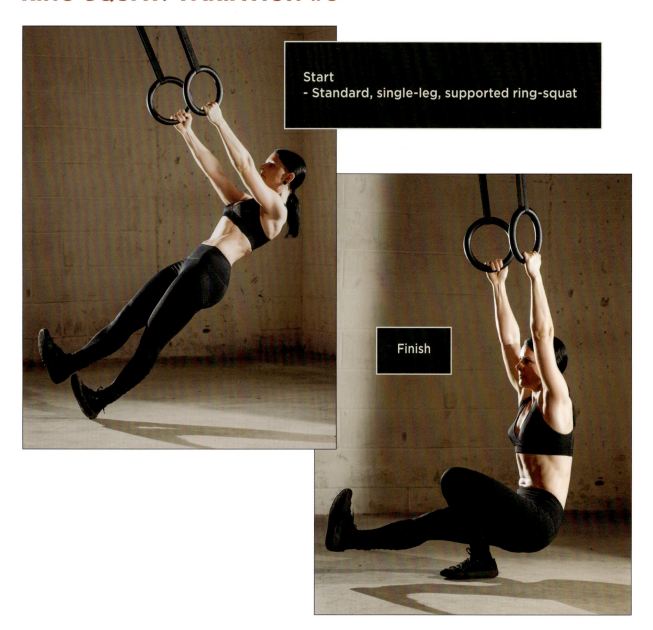

Start
- Standard, single-leg, supported ring-squat

Finish

RING DIP POINTS-OF-PERFORMANCE:

- Keep shins oriented vertically
- Arms are straight and relaxed
- Weight is on the heels
- Squat down, not back
- Squat past 180 degrees for a legit rep
- Get tight before the descent (especially when on one leg) and lower yourself with control

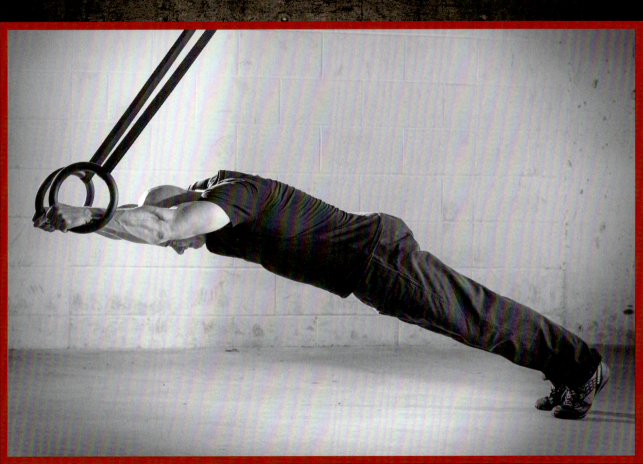

TRUNK EXTENSION
– RING ROLL-OUTS –

SET-UP

Ring roll-outs are named because they mimic the forward "roll out" movement of the ab-wheel. But unlike an ab-wheel, the rings offer many more options for the user to adjust the difficulty of the exercise.

The rings will need to be set low to the floor for ring roll-outs. But keep in mind that the lower the rings, the more difficult the exercise will be to perform. You will also need to demonstrate complete control of overall body tension—from head to toe. If you lose control during the easier variations, you might only fall to your knees. But if you can't stay tight during variations #2 or #3, you may find yourself falling face-first onto the floor. So don't rush this exercise, control is key.

When grasping the rings for ring roll-outs, the palms face towards each other rather than towards the floor. It may help to think of punching forward with a vertical fist. This will keep the bones of the arm aligned and reduce stress on the wrists and elbows. As you "roll" forward it is imperative to keep the arms straight and locked in place. As you continue forward, imagine that your midsection is under tension, like a rubber band. The closer your midsection gets to the floor, imagine that band is being pulled tighter and tighter. At the bottom of the movement, when you have "flattened out", allow that stored muscle-tension to release, pulling you back in and up, completing the repetition.

RING ROLL-OUT: VARIATION #1

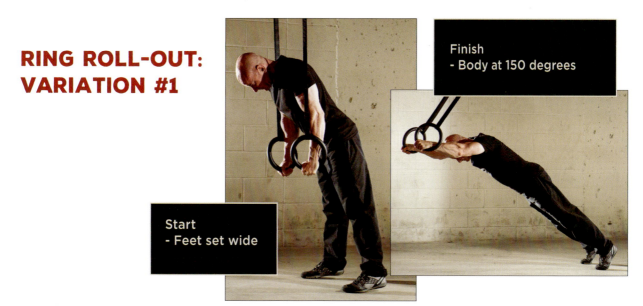

Finish
- Body at 150 degrees

Start
- Feet set wide

RING ROLL-OUT: VARIATION #2

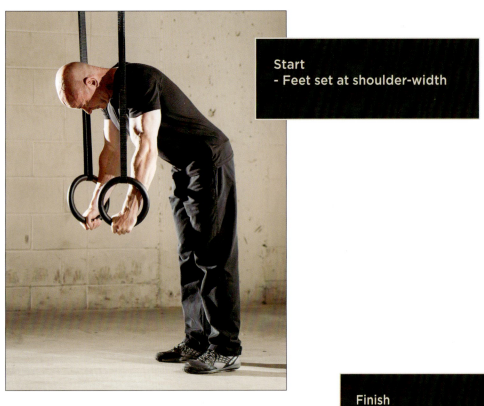

Start
- Feet set at shoulder-width

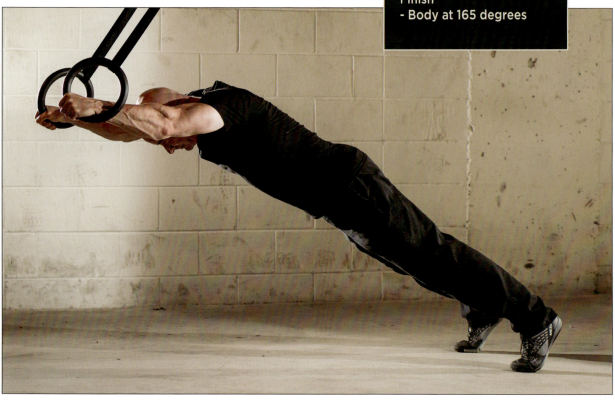

Finish
- Body at 165 degrees

RING ROLL-OUT: VARIATION #3

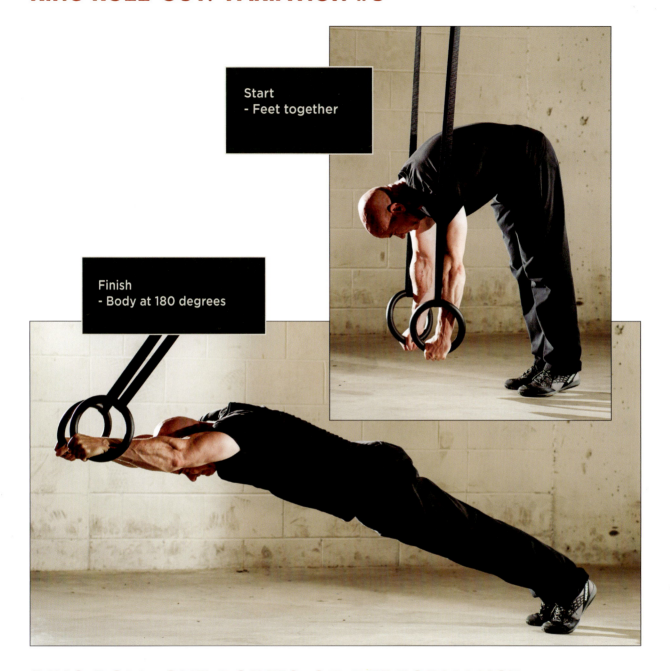

Start
- Feet together

Finish
- Body at 180 degrees

RING ROLL-OUT POINTS-OF-PERFORMANCE:

- Palms face inward
- Arms are straight and locked
- Arms stay in line with the trunk
- Shoulders stay snug in their sockets
- Descend under control
- Create waist-down tension by contracting the glutes, legs and toes

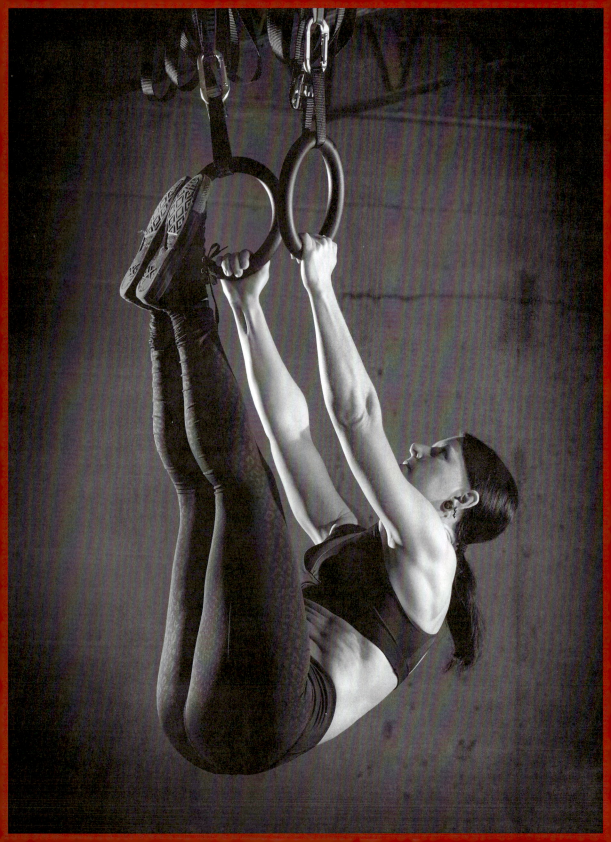

TRUNK FLEXION
– RING RAISES –

SET-UP

Ring raises emphasize the abdominal muscles and hip-flexors. They are a more athletically-oriented midsection movement than most commonly performed ground-based exercises. They are a challenging exercise and seldom seen outside of a gymnastics studio.

The gymnast variation of this exercise is typically performed on a horizontal bar and is very precise in both posture and tempo. Posture-wise, gymnasts cultivate what is called a hollow position which entails a flattening of the lower back and pulling the chest forward. While this is a foundational posture for more advanced gymnastics skills, it does not relate to our purely strength-centric objectives. The body position for ring raises is more "spine-neutral", since the rings allow the body to move further backward as a unit reducing the compressive effects of the hollow position as the legs reach the apex of the movement.

In terms of tempo, a gymnast performs leg raises at a slow to medium tempo. Part of the gymnast's objective is activating the abdominals and hip-flexors by raising their legs towards the bar. Their other objective is to do this while maintaining their hollow position. The gymnast has a dual goal of building strength as well as reinforcing technique.

The other variable which makes ring raises different from their straight bar counterparts is the pendulum-esque nature of the rings. A fixed straight bar gives you something to swing against, but the rings can seem to have a mind of their own during ring raises. One way to manage this is by limiting the amount of space between the anchor point and the rings themselves. The longer the length of webbing, the more potential pendulum-motion you will introduce into the exercise.

RING RAISES: VARIATION #1

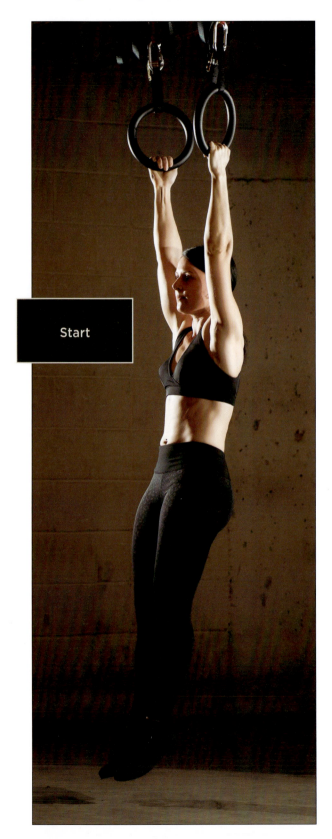

Start

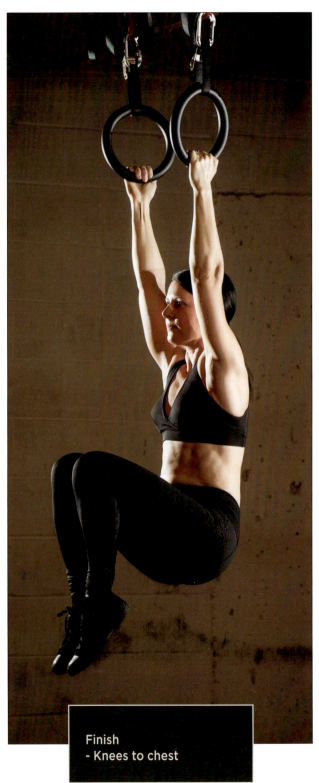

Finish
- Knees to chest

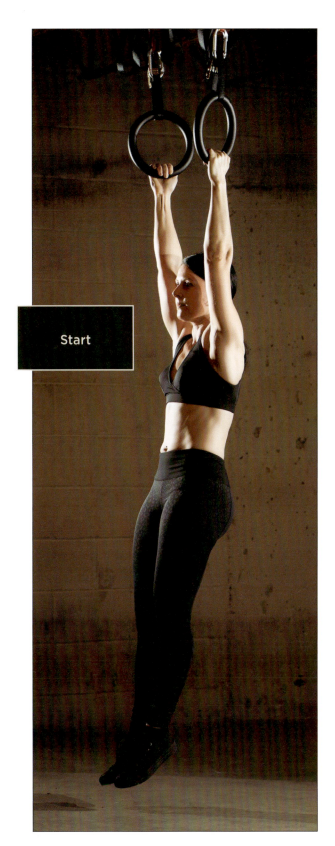
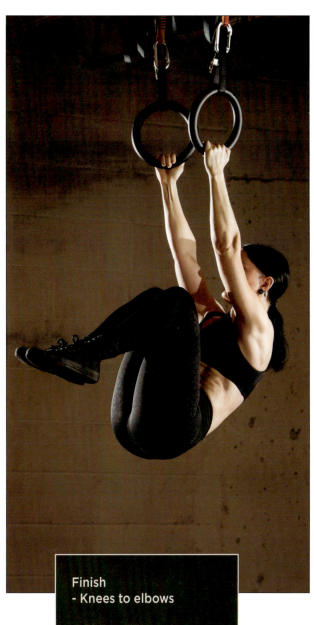

RING RAISES: VARIATION #3

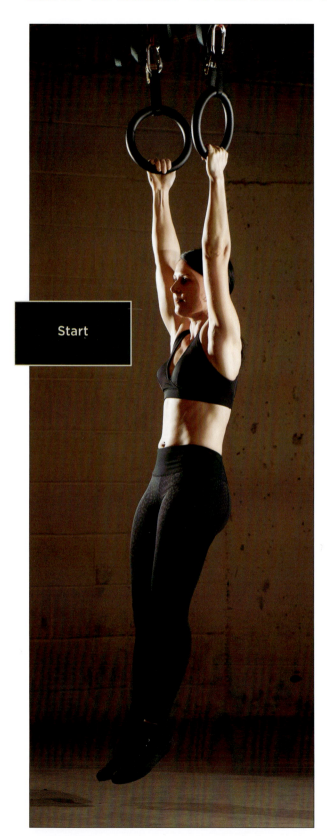

Start

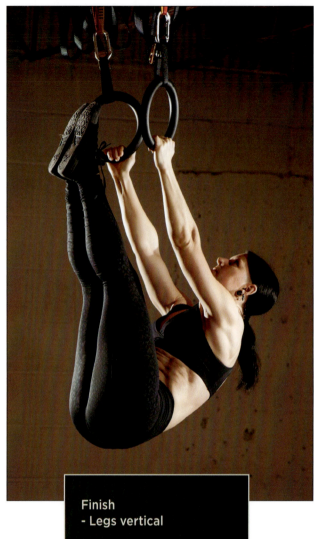

Finish
- Legs vertical

RING RAISE POINTS-OF-PERFORMANCE:

- Rings are set shoulder-width apart
- Grasp rings with an overhand grip
- Avoid excessive swing
- Raise the legs with muscle power, not momentum

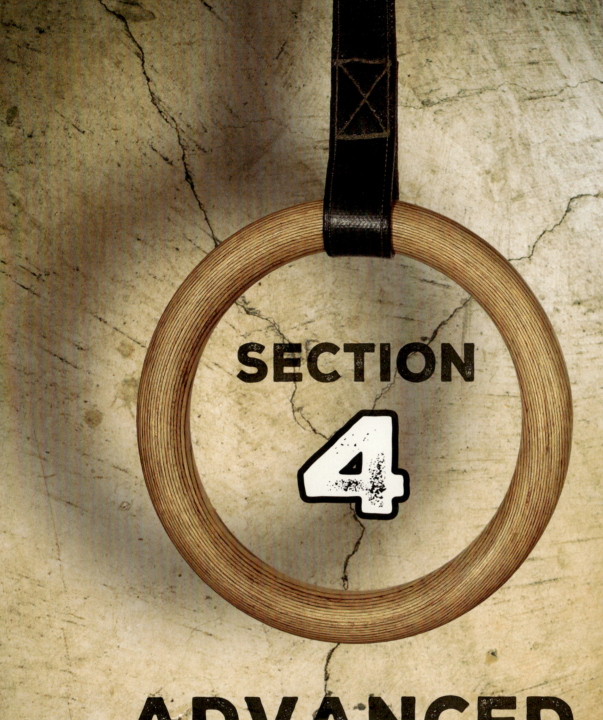

SECTION 4

ADVANCED RING CONCEPTS

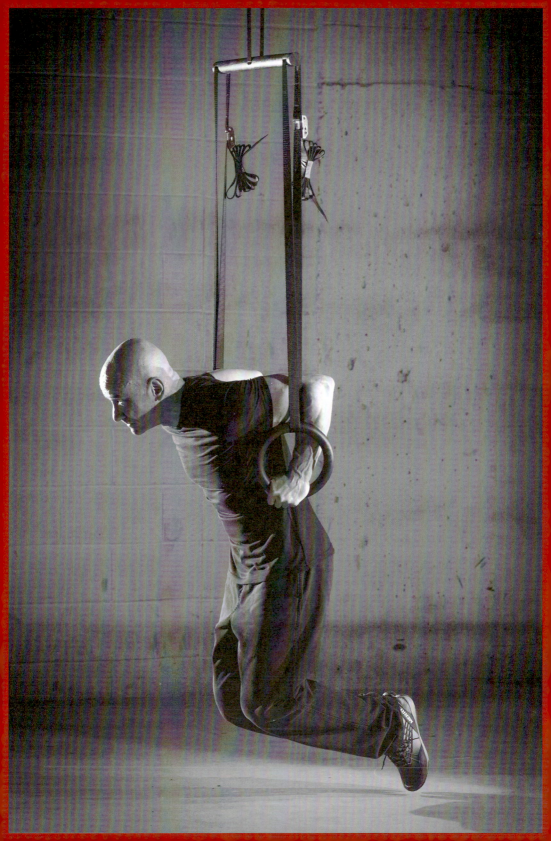

FINESSING FORM WITH THE 'WOBBLE BAR'

This section will introduce you to an exciting evolution in ring training; the "Wobble Bar". I first arrived at the idea of the Wobble Bar in 2012, after I began working with a high-level gymnastics club. Because my athletes adapted so quickly to ring training, I wanted to find a way to continue to challenge their strength levels while simultaneously improving the quality of their ring movements. These gymnasts were subsequently exposed to several versions of the Wobble Bar, but they were the only ones. Then, during my initial discussions with John Du Cane about the topic of ring training, I shared the Wobble Bar concept with him. We decided that **Rings of Power** would provide the perfect vehicle to introduce this invaluable ring training accessory to the rest of the world.

The Wobble Bar provides the proverbial "next level" of ring training. It does this is by discouraging poor exercise technique. When you perform work on rings suspended from a Wobble Bar, you will receive immediate user feedback. If your form is clean and your body is tight, you are rewarded by a stable platform from which to work. But if you try and get by with sloppy repetitions the bar will penalize you by either rocking you back and forth (oscillation) or spinning you in circles (rotation). Any issues of low body tension or poor form become self-correcting.

In addition to improving the technique of a given exercise, the Wobble Bar also provides the means to identify unilateral weakness. If one side of the user's body is weaker than the other, consistent use of the Wobble Bar will provide a swift resolution to these muscular imbalances.

The Wobble Bar is designed to be used with the upper-body pulling and pushing progressions. Specifically, the ring push-up, ring dip, ring-row and ring pull-up. The best way to introduce yourself to the unique rigors of the Wobble Bar is to practice stabilizing yourself in the starting position of the above four exercises. Once you can hold those positions steady, you are ready to proceed. But be aware that even seasoned ring trainers have found the Wobble Bar to be a challenge to conquer. Prepare to take a step back as you lay the groundwork for taking several steps further forward.

SETTING UP THE WOBBLE BAR

Ensure that you create enough "headspace" between the rings and the bar. If headspace is lacking during ring dips, ring pull-ups or ring push-ups, it is very easy to run your head directly into the bar. So set up the Wobble Bar and rings safely by leaving yourself sufficient room to work.

WOBBLE BAR RING PUSH-UP

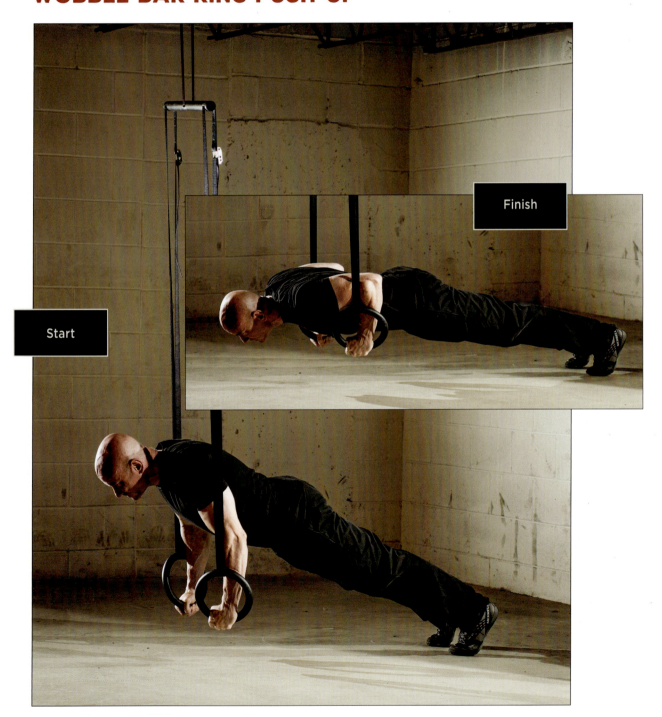

WOBBLE BAR RING DIP

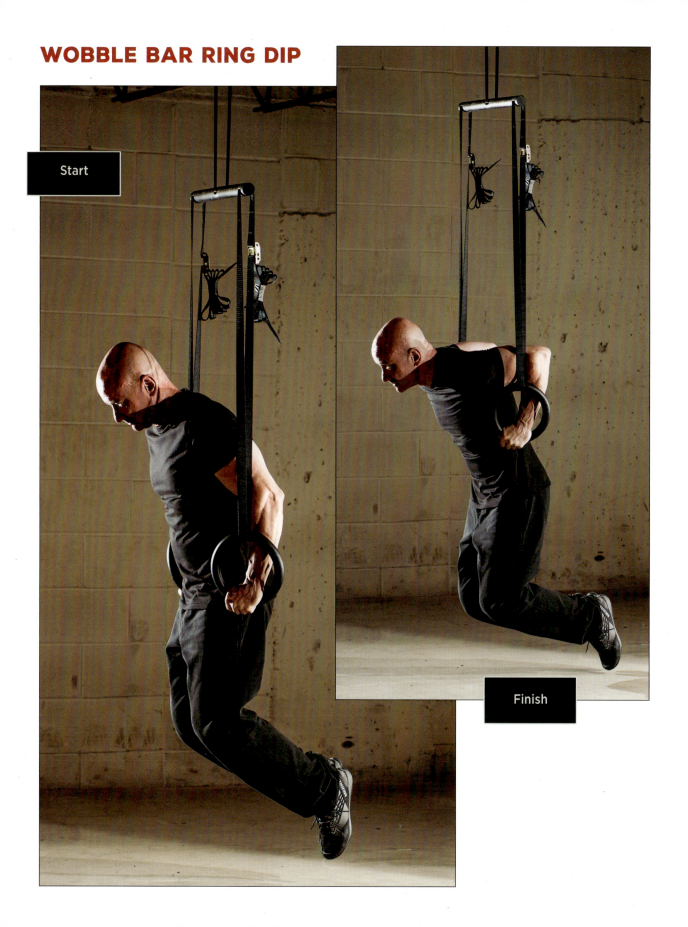

Start

Finish

WOBBLE BAR RING ROW

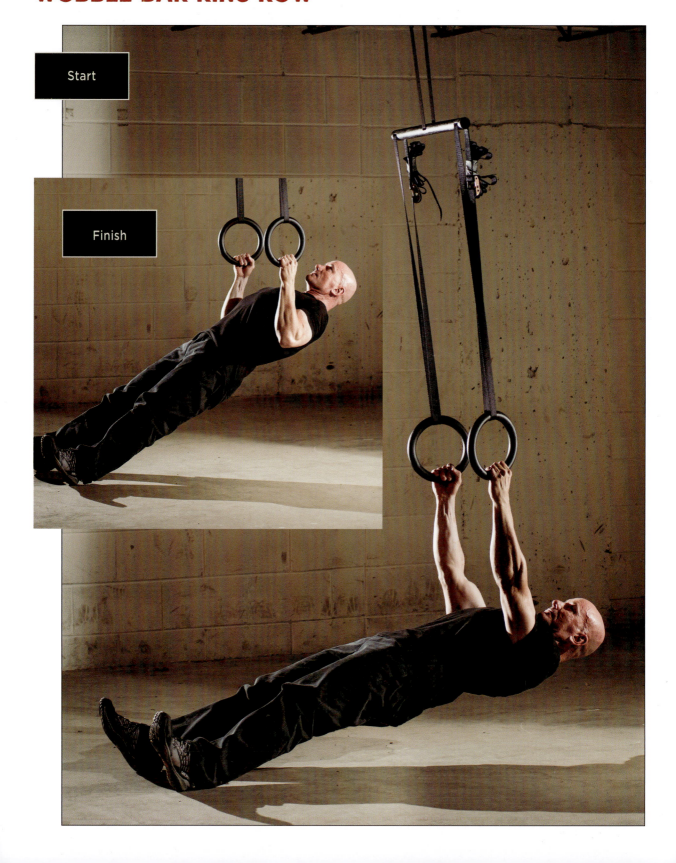

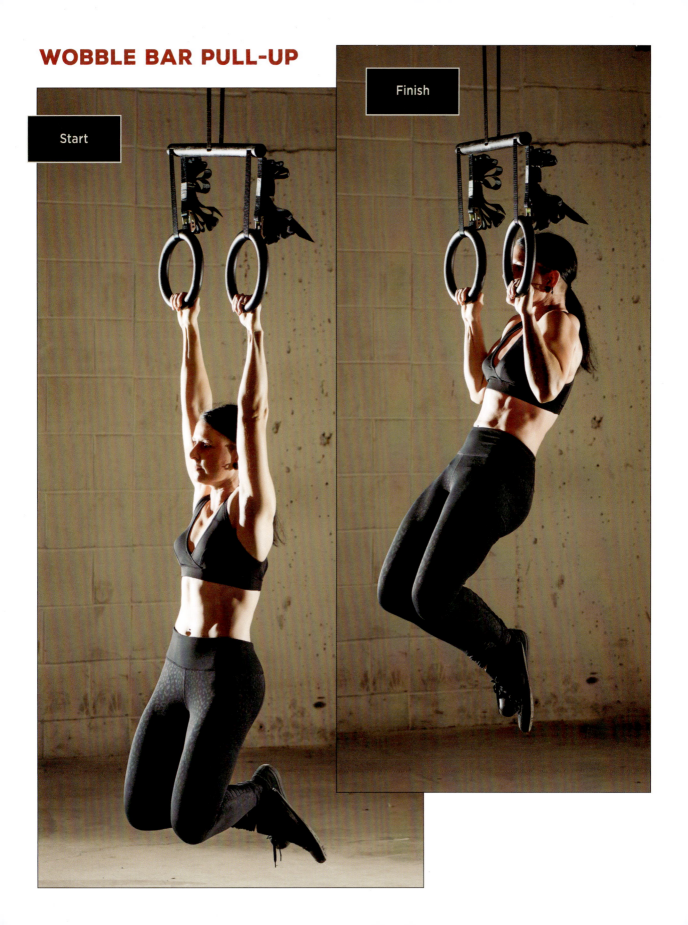

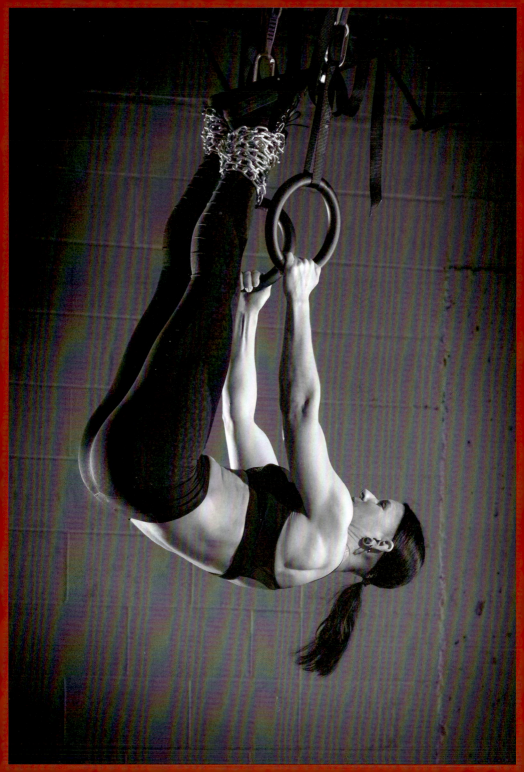

INVERTED RING PROGRESSIONS

These inverted progressions provide additional opportunities for both challenge and variety in your strength training. Variety is a particularly valuable variable to inject into your strength regimen. When repeatedly exposed to the same training stimulus, your body eventually becomes accustomed to that stressor. This means that your body—a perpetually adaptive organism—is no longer "stressed" by that particular stressor. It no longer has to adapt to this new norm. This is when progress can flat line. So the sheer variety of movement patterns provided by ring training is a most effective way to keep your body adapting and becoming stronger.

The other benefit of having an array of angle options is that eventually, something will hurt. It is an inevitability of training that a particular movement will become uncomfortable to perform. The solution is to find a "work-around", something that provides an effective alternative for targeting a desired movement pattern or muscle group. At these times, the highly mobile and adjustable nature of rings make them a uniquely "therapeutic" strength tool.

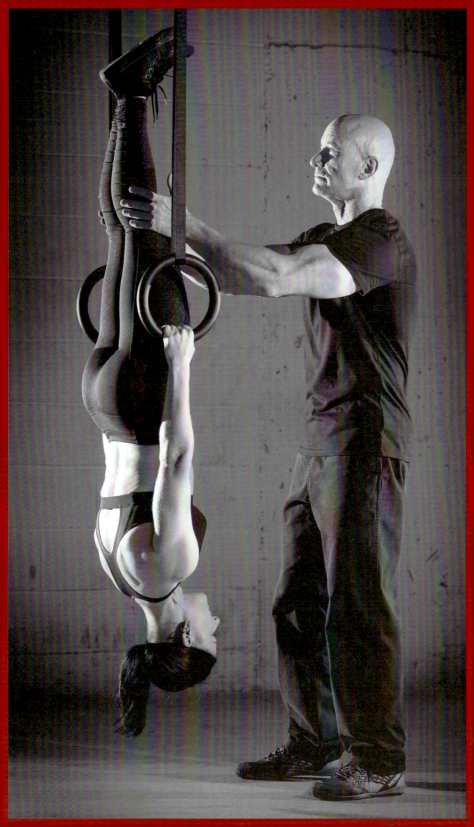

VERTICAL PULLING
– INVERTED RING PULL-UPS –

SET-UP

When prepping the rings for inverted ring pull-ups, you will need to allow for your legs being above you rather than below you. While this may seem obvious, this movement requires a good deal more overhead clearance than the other progressions.

For many people, one of the big challenges associated with this movement is psychological rather than physical. Being upside down is an unfamiliar feeling and people will often feel "out of control" when they first invert themselves. This can cause a brief sense of panic leading to flailing legs in an effort to "find the floor" for get right-side-up again. Unfortunately, some people give up on this position before they ever really get started. But in actuality, the inverted position is not that difficult to hold.

Even if you never progress to performing inverted ring pull-ups, just learning to maintain the inverted position is a very valuable core exercise. If you start on this movement by working with a spotter, you can find yourself getting comfortable with the position very quickly.

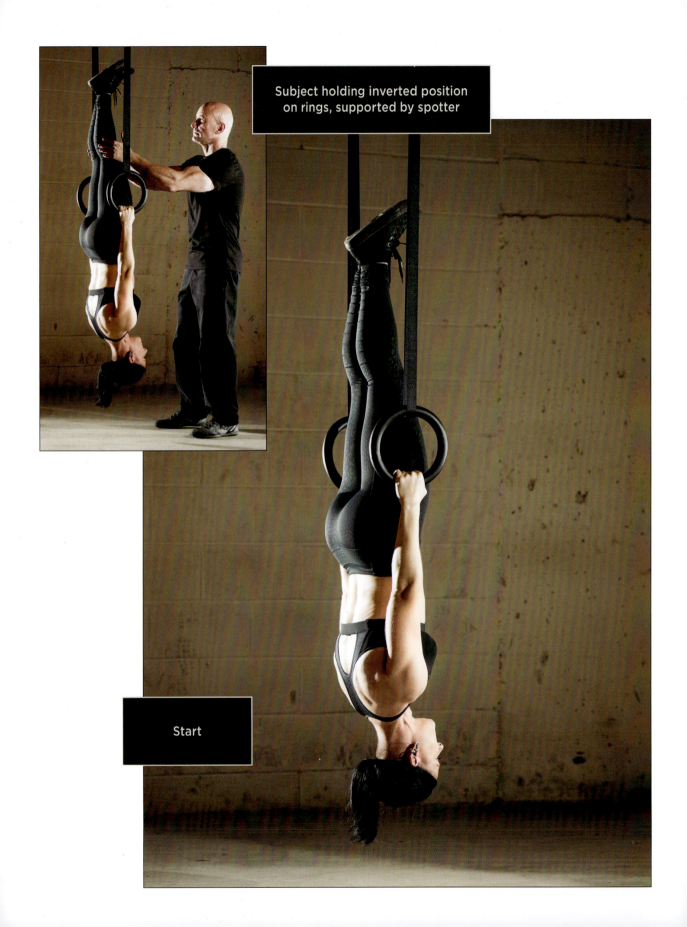

Subject holding inverted position on rings, supported by spotter

Start

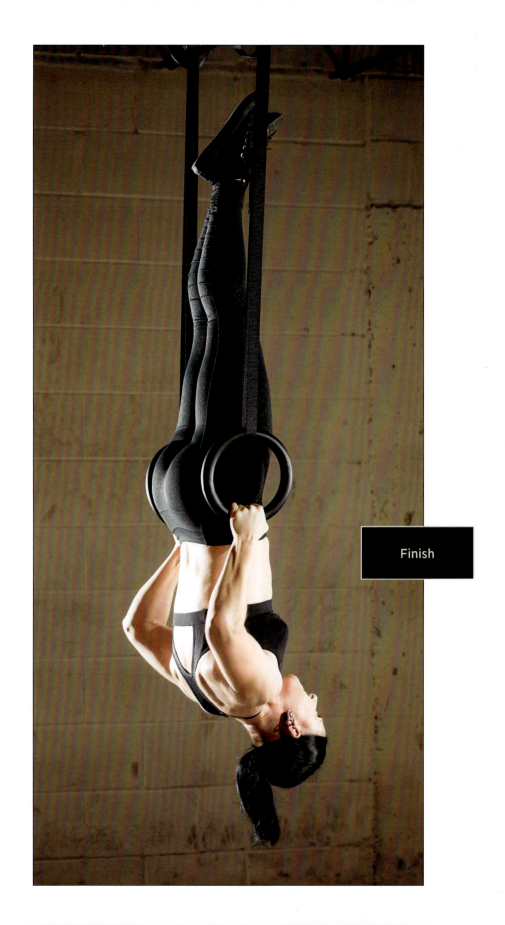

Finish

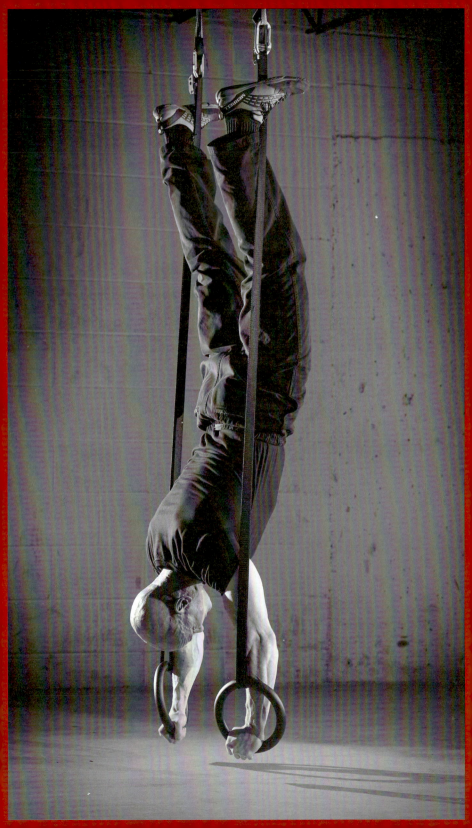

VERTICAL PUSHING
– INVERTED RING PUSH-UPS –

SET-UP

Setting up the rings for inverted ring push-ups must take into account where your head will go while in the "down" position. Set the rings low, but not so low that your head makes contact with floor prior to completing the movement.

Understand that the final variation of this movement is the most difficult exercise in this book. It is also the most dangerous—especially if you are either not ready for it or not paying 100% attention during its execution. It is strongly advised that you do not try the completely inverted, unsupported variation until you have performed a number of successful repetitions with a spotter. Like heavy deadlifts or back squats, the most beneficial exercises can also be the riskiest. *This exercise is no exception.* Do not attempt it until you have earned the right to do so.

INVERTED RING PUSH-UPS: VARIATION #1

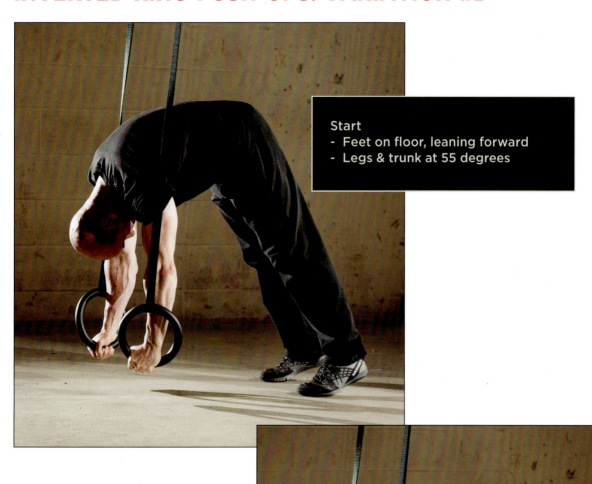

Start
- Feet on floor, leaning forward
- Legs & trunk at 55 degrees

Finish

INVERTED RING PUSH-UPS: VARIATION #2

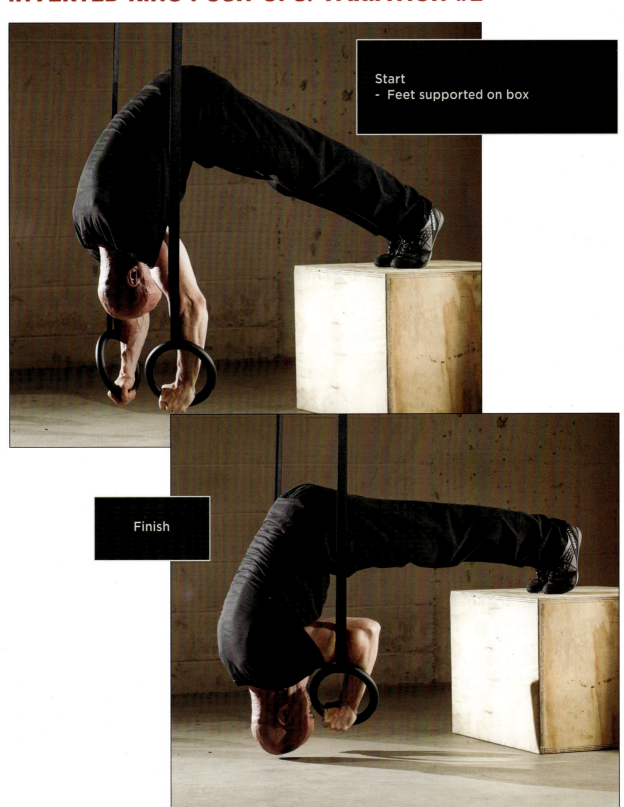

Start
- Feet supported on box

Finish

INVERTED RING PUSH-UPS: VARIATION #3

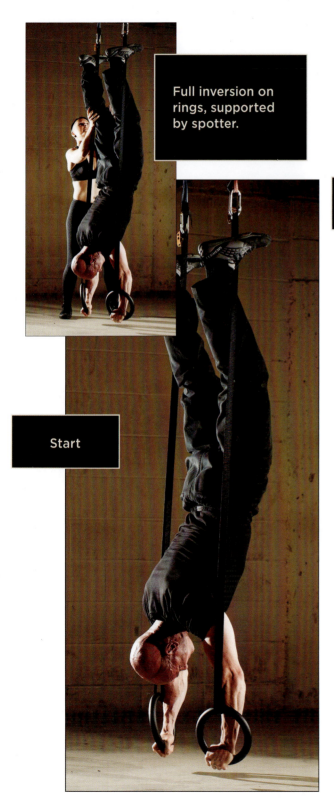

Start

Full inversion on rings, supported by spotter.

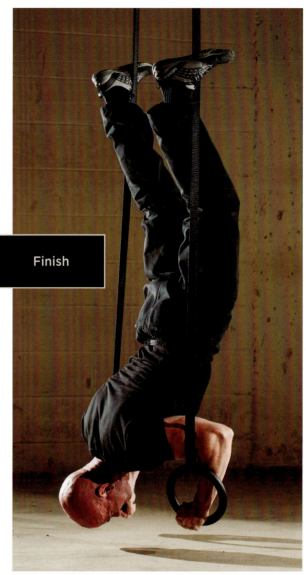

Finish

INVERTED RING PUSH-UP POINTS-OF-PERFORMANCE:

- Keep the trunk oriented vertically, even during the supported variations
- Keep shoulders "tight" in their sockets
- Control your descent, don't hit your head on the floor
- If you haven't mastered unsupported ring dips do not attempt unsupported inverted ring push-ups

EXTERNAL LOADING

Consistent application of technique and tenacity in the performance of the seven primary movement patterns in this book will build substantial levels of strength. But the serious strength-seeker is always looking ahead for the next challenge. If you were harboring any concerns that you might one day become too strong for ring training, let me put those fears to rest right now.

The good news is that each of the seven primary movement patterns can be further enhanced through external loading. This simply means that by adding additional weight to your body with a weight vest, chains, kettlebells and so on you can perpetually adjust and increase the intensity of these exercises.

There are a number of ways that you can load yourself to increase the resistance of these various movements. For the purposes of this book, the examples will be improvised as opposed to being reliant on specialty equipment such as weight vests. While there are quality vests on the market, they are expensive. My goal is to teach you how to load your body at minimal expense. The reason for this is psychological rather than functional. I don't want you to think that the advanced applications of ring training are out of your reach because of the cost. Be resourceful.

LOADING EXAMPLES

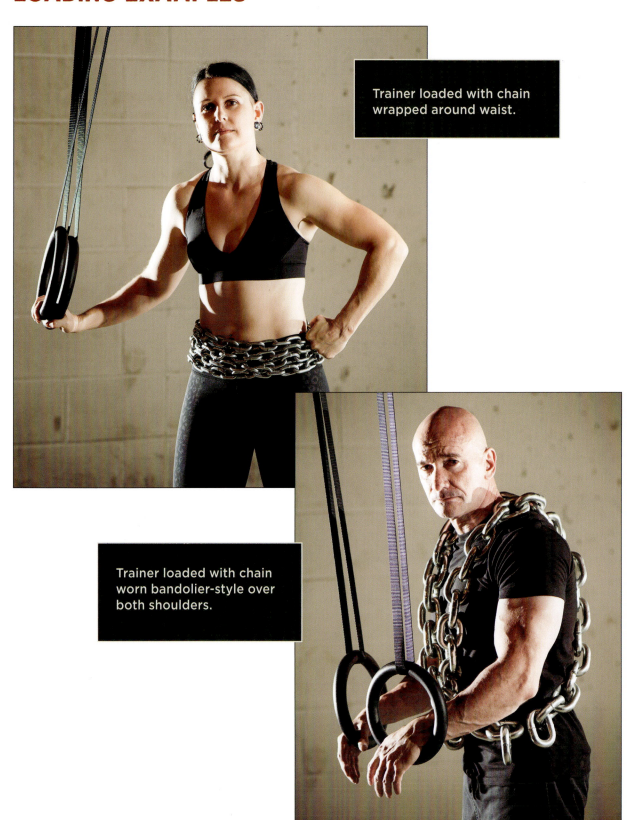

Trainer loaded with chain wrapped around waist.

Trainer loaded with chain worn bandolier-style over both shoulders.

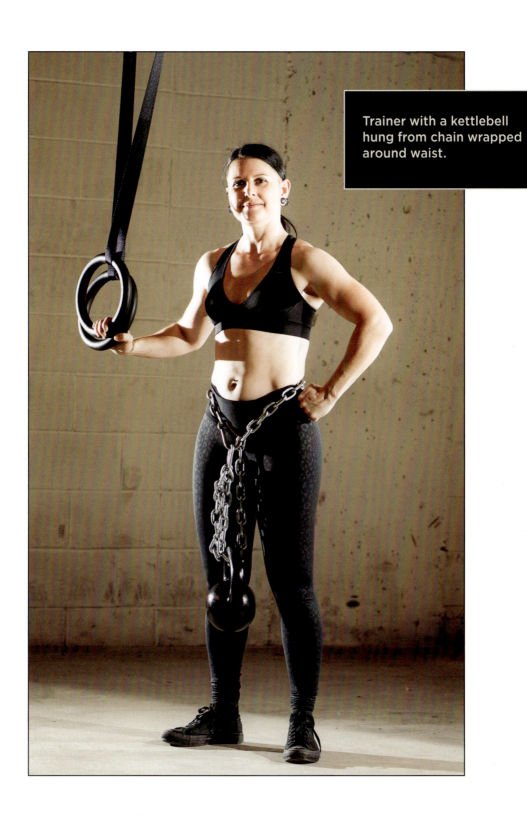

Trainer with a kettlebell hung from chain wrapped around waist.

LOADING EXERCISE EXAMPLES

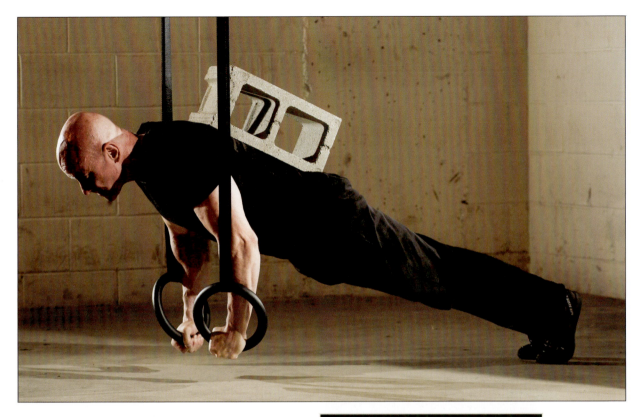

Loading the Ring Push-Up...

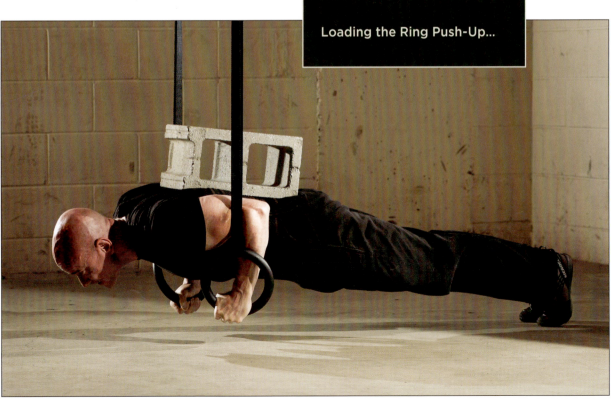

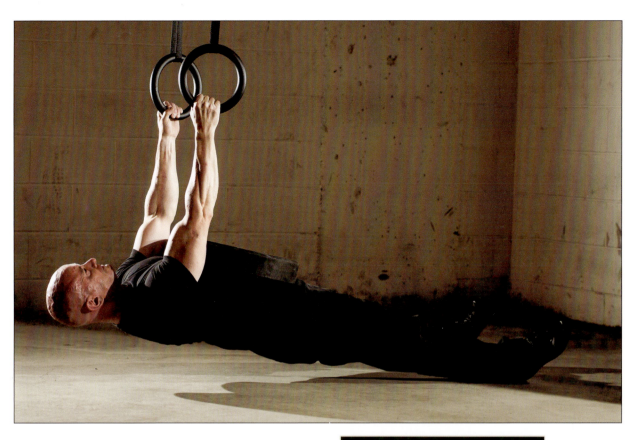

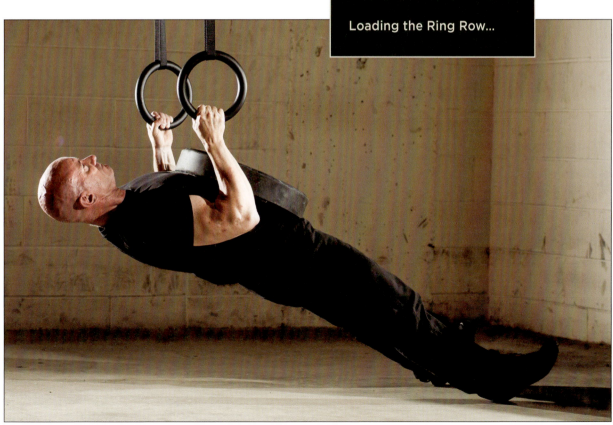

Loading the Ring Row...

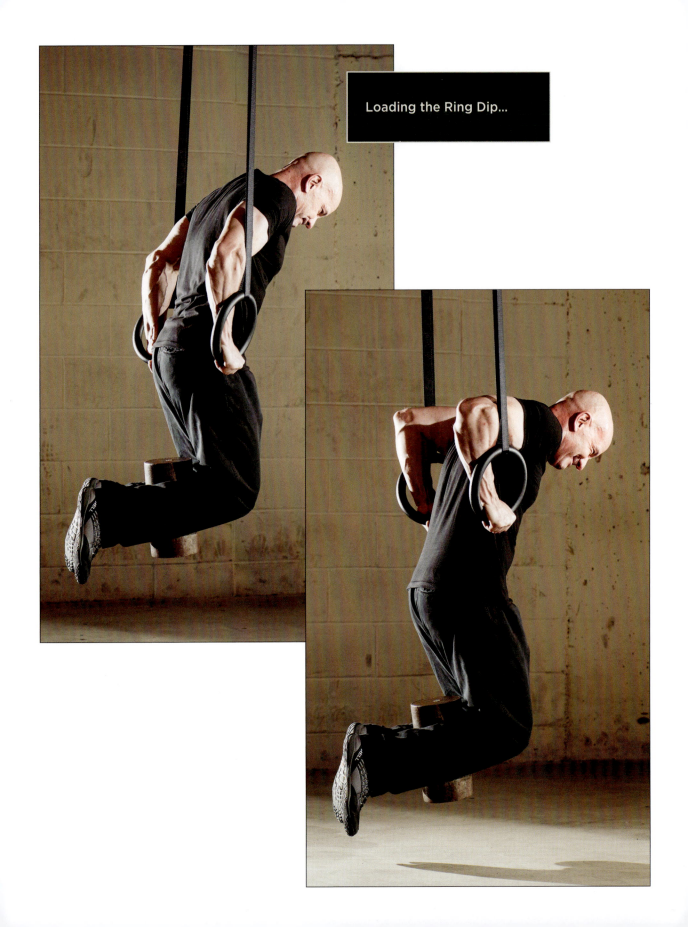

Loading the Ring Dip...

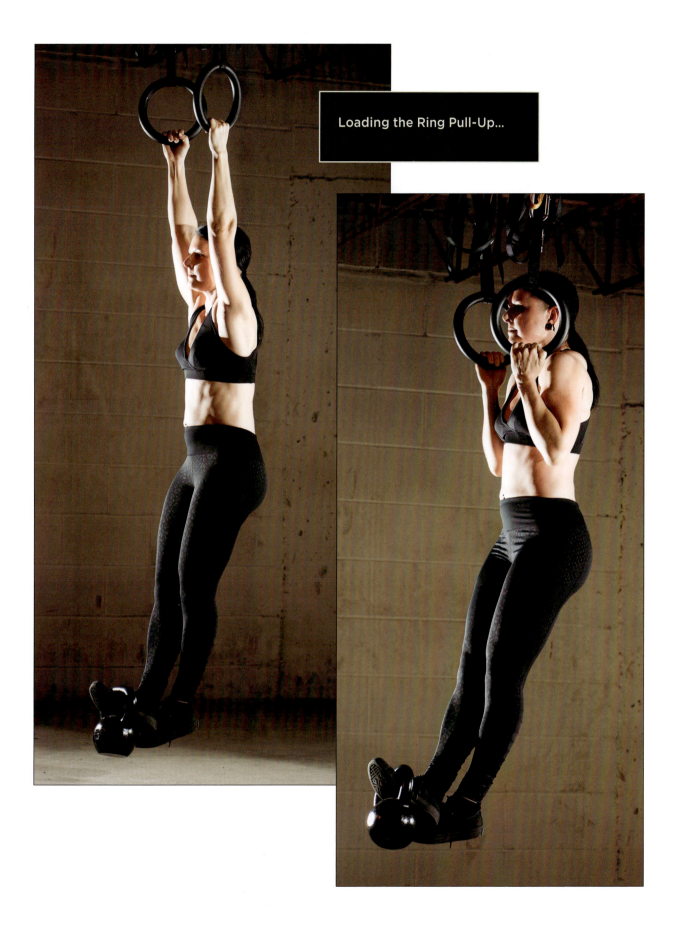

Loading the Ring Pull-Up...

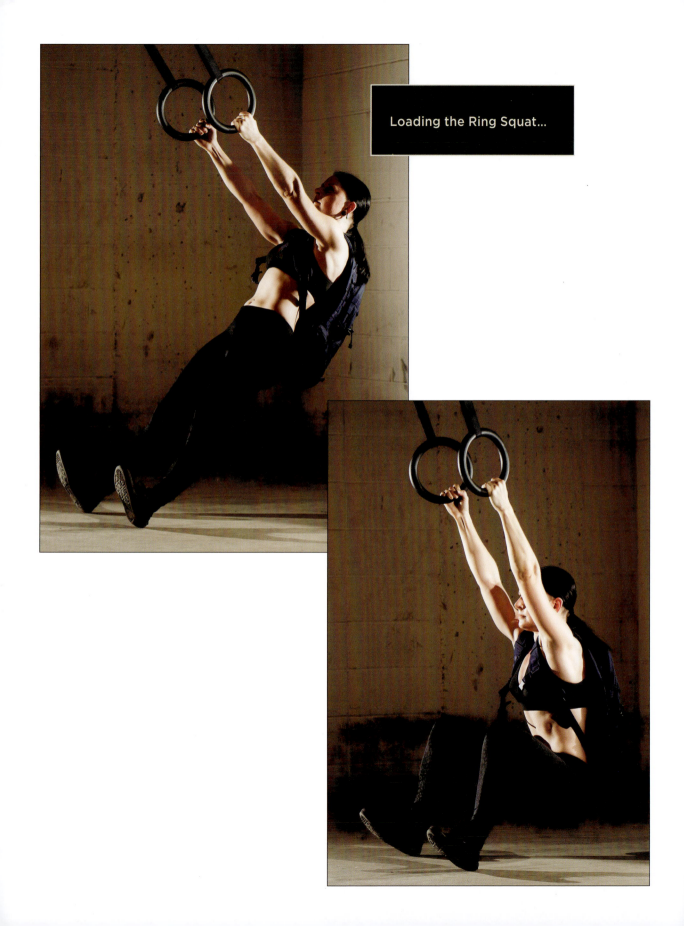

Loading the Ring Squat...

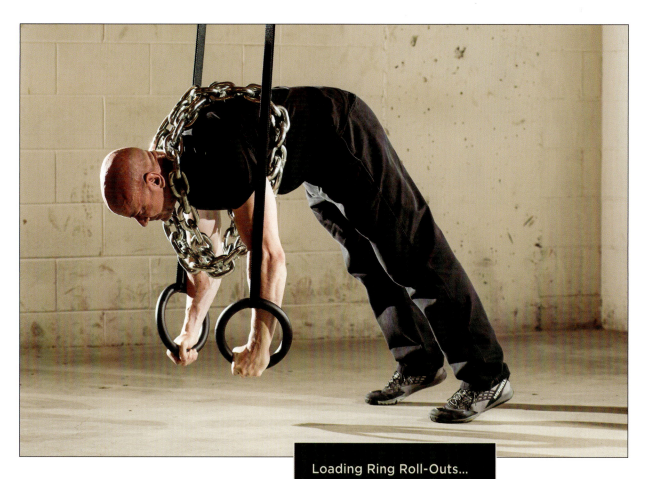

Loading Ring Roll-Outs...

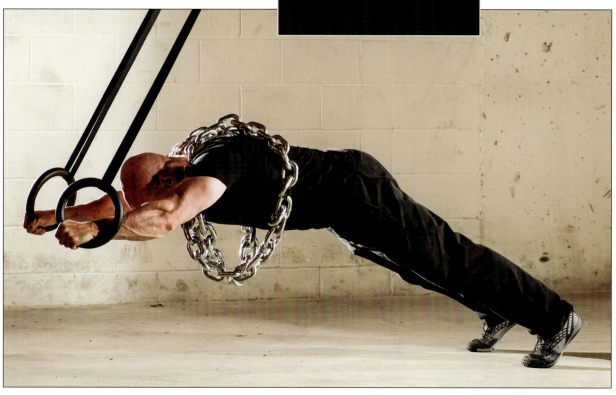

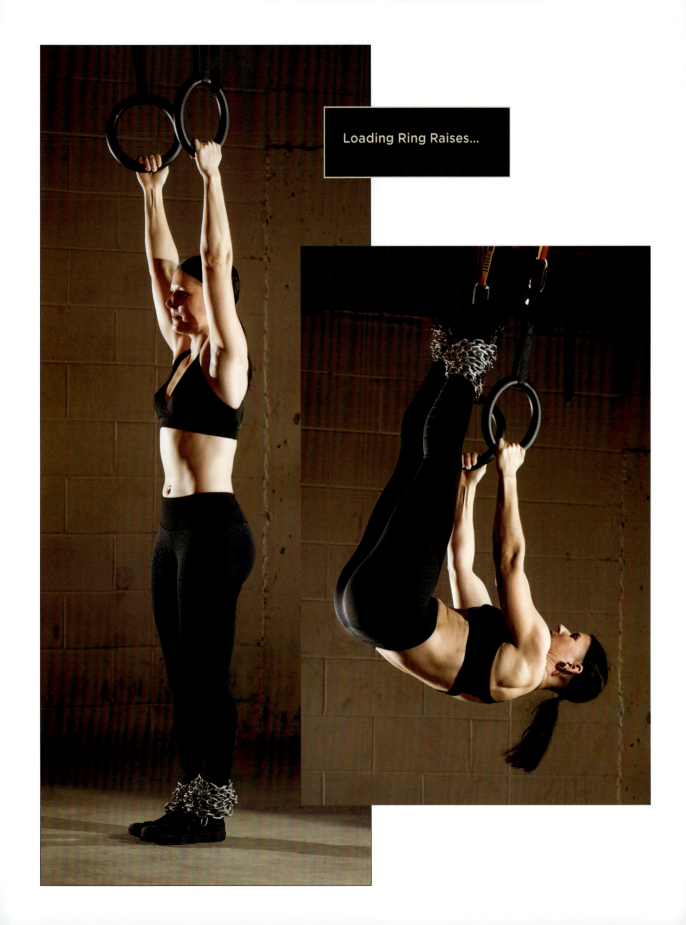

Loading Ring Raises...

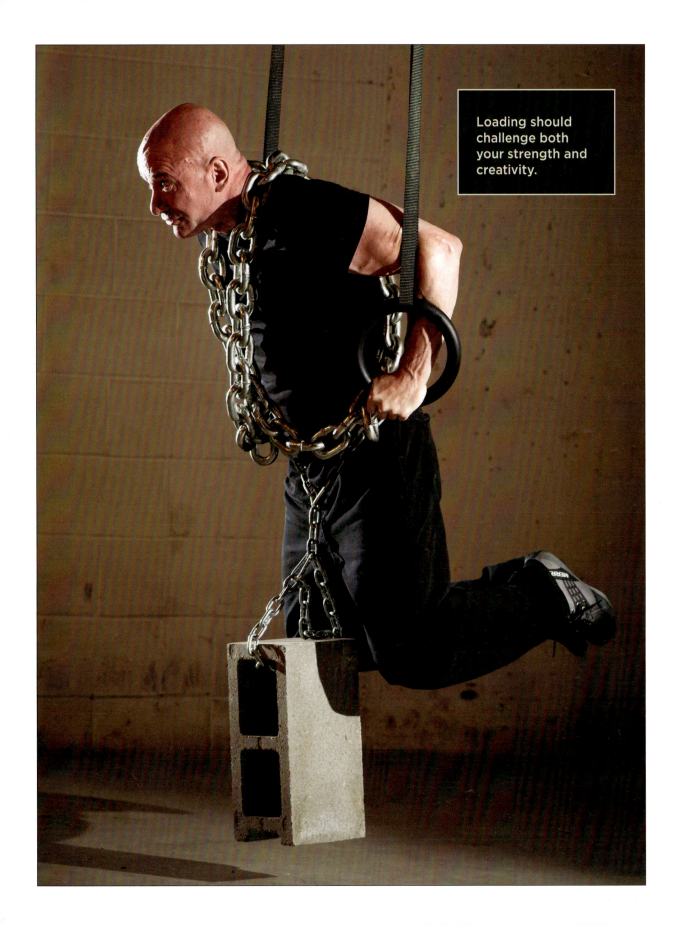

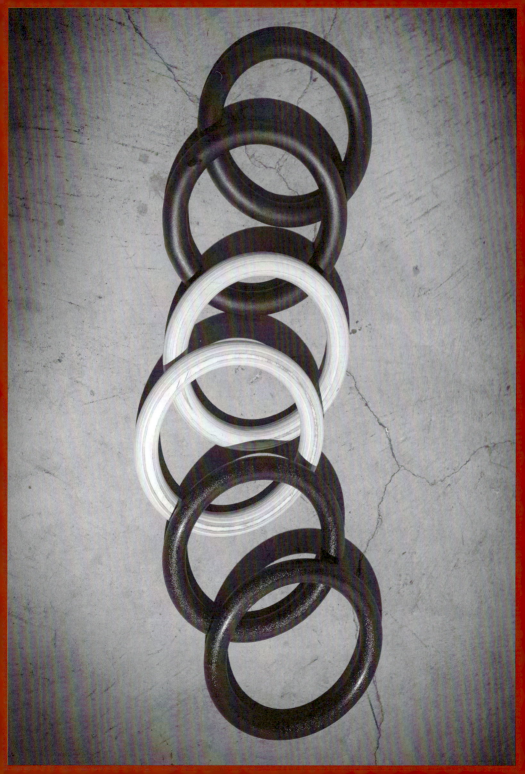

RING WORKOUTS

The most important ring training concept to grasp is that the workout is secondary. It is far more important that you prioritize mastering the movements instead of worrying about sets and reps. As you work to perfect your form on the movements, your strength will improve.

Your immediate goal should be to get to the *variation #3 level* of each movement. Once this has been accomplished, you can then work towards being able to master the Wobble Bar, performing loaded movements, and conquering the inverted variations.

When starting out, remember that you need to begin with the variation you can perform correctly. Do quality work. Progress will not be symmetrical. You will master some progressions sooner than others. Once you get to the point where you can do some repetitions of a "standard" variation, it is fine to combine one standard set with several subsequent sets of an easier version of the same exercise. As long as you remain consistent, you should eventually progress to more the challenging variations of all the exercises.

In general, when pursuing strength, keep the load high and the reps low. Because people tend to think of ring training as bodyweight or calisthenics training, they gravitate towards greater volume (higher reps) instead of greater tension *(higher load)*. You can go either way you prefer, but I am an advocate for following the path of most resistance *(heavy loads)*.

The 3-A-Week Workout is a total-body program which will provide results for most people for a long time. The 4-A-Week Workout is for those trainees who want to add more variety and volume to their training. It is up to you to employ good judgment and begin your training at your current level, and with your own goals in mind.

RING WORKOUT SCHEDULES

3-A-WEEK WORKOUT
Ring Push-Ups
Ring Rows
Ring Dips
Ring Pull-Ups
Ring Squats
Ring Roll-Outs
Ring Raises

3X PER WEEK
3-4 sets 6-10 reps
3-4 sets 6-10 reps
3-4 sets 6-10 reps
3-4 sets 6-10 reps
3-4 sets 6-10 reps
3-4 sets 6-10 reps
3-4 sets 6-10 reps

4-A-WEEK WORKOUT

Workout A
Ring Push-Ups
Ring Rows
Ring Dips
Ring Pull-Ups

Workout B
Ring Squats
Ring Roll-Outs
Ring Raises

4X PER WEEK (EX: M/TH & T/F)

M/Th
5 sets 6-10 reps
5 sets 6-10 reps
5 sets 6-10 reps
5 sets 6-10 reps

T/F
5 sets 6-10 reps
5 sets 6-10 reps
5 sets 6-10 reps

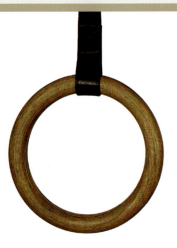
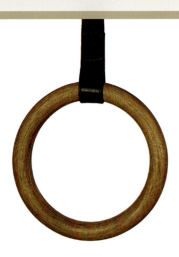

ACKNOWLEDGMENTS

To my Lord and Savior Jesus Christ

To my wife Tammie

To those who have personally inspired me in the ways of physical culture: Dennis Rogers, Patrick Povilaitis, Jon Bruney, Chris Rider, Greg Matonick, Slim "The Hammerman" Farman and Mike Greenstein

To John Du Cane for making this project possible

To Don Pitlik for the amazing photographs

To Adrienne Harvey for sharing her strength in so many of these photographs

To Derek Brigham for the incredible design work

To Dan John for writing the forword

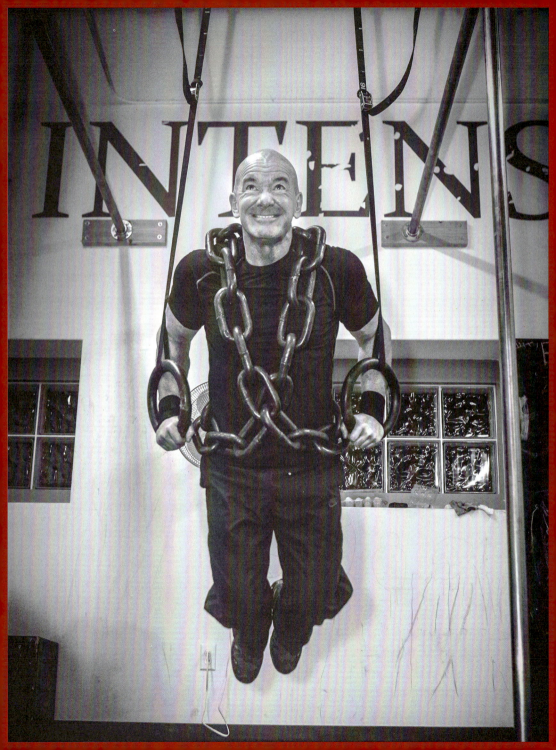

ABOUT THE AUTHOR

Mike Gillette is a life-long seeker of strength in all of its forms. As an end-user, Mike has explored strength-development through the prisms of military service, law enforcement, the martial arts and executive protection. As a performance coach, he has worked with tactical operators, competitive fighters and D1 athletes.

Mike is also a practitioner of feats of mind and body strength and has had several of his unique achievements acknowledged by Guinness World Records and Ripley's Believe it or Not. Mike's blog (www.MikeGillette.com) is a sought-after source of insights and inspiration for all serious students of strength.

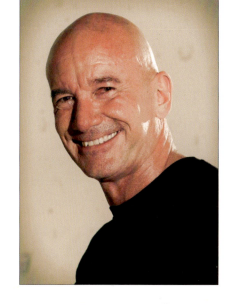

Outside the worlds of physical culture and mental maximization, Mike is a husband, father and grandfather. A self-described music snob and movie buff, his prized possession is a small glass bottle containing some hair from the late Joseph L. Greenstein, better known as "The Mighty Atom", considered to be the greatest strongman who ever lived. A bottle which was presented to Mike at Coney Island, by Greenstein's protégé, Slim "The Hammerman" Farman.

Get Your Ultimate Blueprint for the Attainment of Power, Functional Speed and Agility…

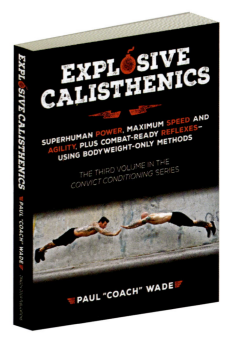

"The first physical attribute we lose as we age is our ability to generate power. Close behind is the loss of skilled, coordinated movement. The fix is never to lose these abilities in the first place! Paul Wade's *Explosive Calisthenics* is the best program for developing power and skilled movement I have seen. Just as with his previous two books, the progressions are masterful with no fancy equipment needed.

Do yourself a favor and get this amazing work. This book will be the gold standard for developing bodyweight power, skill, and agility."
—**Chris Hardy**, D.O. MPH, CSCS, author, **Strong Medicine**

"*Explosive Calisthenics* is an absolute Treasure Map for anybody looking to tear down their body's athletic limitations. Who doesn't want to be able to kip to their feet from their back like a Bruce Lee? Or make a backflip look easy? Paul makes you want to put down the barbells, learn and practice these step-by-step progressions to mastering the most explosive and impressive bodyweight movements. The best part is? You can become an absolute Beast in under an hour of practice a week. Way to go, Paul! AROO!"
—**Joe Distefano, Spartan Race,** Director of Training & Creator of the **Spartan SGX Certification**

"*Explosive Calisthenics* is a masterfully constructed roadmap for the attainment of power, functional speed, and agility."
—**Patrick Roth, M.D.**, author of **The End of Back Pain: Access Your Hidden Core to Heal Your Body**

"Coach Wade saved the best for last! *Explosive Calisthenics* is the book all diehard **Convict Conditioning** fans have been waiting for. There has never been anything like it until now!

With his trademark blend of old-school philosophy, hard-earned wisdom and in-your-face humor, Coach expands his infamous system of progressive bodyweight programming to break down the most coveted explosive moves, including the back flip, kip-up and muscle-up. If you want to know how far you can go training with just your own bodyweight, you owe it to yourself to get this book!"
—**Al Kavadlo**, author, **Stretching Your Boundaries**

Explosive Calisthenics
Superhuman Power, Maximum Speed and Agility, Plus Combat-Ready Reflexes—Using Bodyweight-Only Methods
By Paul "Coach" Wade
#B80 $39.95
eBook $19.95
Paperback 8.5 x 11 392 pages

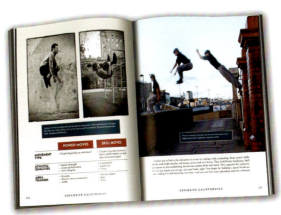

Order Explosive Calisthenics online:
www.dragondoor.com/B80

24 HOURS A DAY ORDER NOW 1•800•899•5111
Visit: www.dragondoor.com

How Do YOU Stack Up Against These 6 Signs of a TRUE Physical Specimen?

According to Paul Wade's Convict Conditioning you earn the right to call yourself a 'true physical specimen' if you can perform the following:

1. AT LEAST one set of 5 one-arm pushups each side—with the ELITE goal of 100 sets each side
2. AT LEAST one set of 5 one-leg squats each side—with the ELITE goal of 2 sets of 50 each side
3. AT LEAST a single one-arm pullup each side—with the ELITE goal of 2 sets of 6 each side
4. AT LEAST one set of 5 hanging straight leg raises—with the ELITE goal of 2 sets of 30
5. AT LEAST one stand-to-stand bridge—with the ELITE goal of 2 sets of 30

Well, how DO you stack up?

hances are that whatever athletic level you have achieved, there are some serious gaps in your OVERALL strength program. Gaps that stop you short of being able to claim status as a truly accomplished strength athlete.

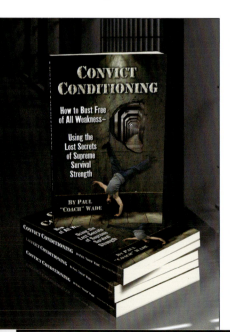

The good news is that—in *Convict Conditioning*—Paul Wade has laid out a brilliant 6-set system of 10 progressions which allows you to master these elite levels.

And you could be starting at almost any age and in almost in any condition...

Paul Wade has given you the keys—ALL the keys you'll ever need— that will open door, after door, after door for you in your quest for supreme physical excellence. Yes, it will be the hardest work you'll ever have to do. And yes, 97% of those who pick up *Convict Conditioning*, frankly, won't have the guts and the fortitude to make it. But if you make it even half-way through **Paul's Progressions**, you'll be stronger than almost anyone you encounter. Ever.

Here's just a small taste of what you'll get with Convict Conditioning:

Can you meet these 5 benchmarks of the *truly* powerful?... Page 1

The nature and the art of real strength... Page 2

Why mastery of *progressive calisthenics* is the ultimate secret for building maximum raw strength... Page 2

A dozen one-arm handstand pushups without support—anyone? Anyone?... Page 3

How to rank in a powerlifting championship—*without ever training with weights*... Page 4

Calisthenics as a hardcore strength training technology... Page 9

Spartan "300" calisthenics at the Battle of Thermopolylae... Page 10

How to cultivate the perfect body—the Greek and Roman way... Page 10

The difference between "old school" and "new school" calisthenics... Page 15

The role of prisons in preserving the older systems... Page 16

Strength training as a primary survival strategy... Page 16

The 6 basic benefits of bodyweight training... Pages 22—27

Why calisthenics are the *ultimate* in functional training... Page 23

The value of cultivating *self-movement*—rather than *object-movement*... Page 23

The *real* source of strength—it's not your *muscles*... Page 24

One crucial reason why a lot of convicts deliberately avoid weight-training... Page 24

How to progressively strengthen your joints over a lifetime—and even heal old joint injuries... Page 25

Why "authentic" exercises like pullups are so perfect for strength and power development... Page 25

Bodyweight training for quick physique perfection... Page 26

How to normalize and regulate your body fat levels—with bodyweight training only... Page 27

Why weight-training and the psychology of overeating go hand in hand... Page 27

The best approach for rapidly strengthening your whole body is this... Page 30

This is the most important and revolutionary feature of *Convict Conditioning*.... Page 33

A jealously-guarded system for going from puny to powerful—when your life may depend on the speed of your results... Page 33

The 6 "Ultimate" Master Steps—only a handful of athletes in the whole world can correctly perform them all. Can you?... Page 33

How to Forge Armor-Plated Pecs and Steel Triceps... Page 41

Why the pushup is the *ultimate* upper body exercise—and better than the bench press... Page 41

How to effectively bulletproof the vulnerable rotator cuff muscles... Page 42

Order Convict Conditioning online: www.dragondoor.com/B41

24 HOURS A DAY ORDER NOW **1-800-899-5111**
Visit: www.dragondoor.com

Observe these 6 important rules for power-packed pushups... Page 42

How basketballs, baseballs and *kissing-the-baby* all translate into greater strength gains... Page 44

How to guarantee steel rod fingers... Page 45

Do you make this stupid mistake with your push ups? This is wrong, wrong, wrong!... Page 45

How to achieve 100 consecutive one-arm pushups each side... Page 64

Going Beyond the One-Arm Pushup... Pages 68—74

Going up!— how to build elevator-cable thighs... Page 75

Where the *real* strength of an athlete lies... Page 75

Most athletic movements rely largely on this attribute... Page 76

The first thing to go as an athlete begins to age—and what you MUST protect... Page 76

THE best way to develop truly powerful, athletic legs... Page 77

The phenomenon of *Lombard's Paradox*—and it contributes to power-packed thighs... Page 78

Why bodyweight squats blow barbell squats away... Page 79

The enormous benefits of mastering the one-leg squat... Page 80

15 secrets to impeccable squatting—for greater power and strength... Pages 81—82

Transform skinny legs into pillars of power, complete with steel cord quads, rock-hard glutes and thick, shapely calves... Page 102

How to achieve one hundred perfect consecutive one-leg squats on each leg... Page 102

Going Beyond the One-Leg Squat... Pages 106—112

How to add conditioning, speed, agility and endurance to legs that are already awesome.... Page 107

How to construct a barn door back—and walk with loaded guns... Page 113

Why our culture has failed to give the pullup the respect and attention it deserves... Page 113

Benefits of the pullup—king of back exercises... Page 114

The dormant superpower for muscle growth waiting to be released if you only do this... Page 114

Why pullups are the single best exercise for building melon-sized biceps... Page 115

Why the pullup is THE safest upper back exercise... Page 115

The single most important factor to consider for your grip choice... Page 118

How to earn lats that look like wings and an upper back sprouting muscles like coiled pythons... Page 138

How to be strong enough to rip a bodybuilder's arm off in an arm wrestling match... Page 138

How to take a trip to hell—and steal a Satanic six-pack... Page 149

The 5 absolute truths that define a genuine six-pack from hell... Page 150

This is the REAL way to gain a six-pack from hell... Page 152

3 big reasons why—in prisons—leg raises have always been much more popular than sit-ups... Page 152

Why the hanging leg raise is the greatest single abdominal exercise known to man... Page 153

10 waist training secrets to help you master the hanging leg raise... Pages 154—155

How to correctly perform the greatest all-round midsection exercise in existence... Page 174

Going beyond the hanging straight leg raise... Page 178

Setting your sights on the most powerful midsection exercise possible—the V raise.... Page 178

How to develop abdominal muscles with enormous contractile power—and iron hip strength... Page 178

How to combat-proof your spine... Page 185

Why the bridge is the most important strength-building exercise in the world... Page 185

How to train your spine—as if your life depended on it... Page 185

Why you should sell your barbell set and buy a cushioned mat instead... Page 188

How to absorb punitive strikes against your spine—and bounce back smiling... Page 188

Why lower back pain is the foremost plague of athletes the world over... Page 189

Why bridging is the *ultimate* exercise for the spinal muscles... Page 189

The 4 signs of the perfect bridge... Page 191

How to master the bridge... Page 192

How to own a spine that feels like a steel whip... Page 193

How the bridging series will grant you an incredible combination of strength paired with flexibility... Page 216

Why bridging stands alone as a *total* training method that facilitates development in practically every area of fitness and health... Page 216

How to look exceptionally masculine—with broad, etched, and powerful shoulders... Page 219

Those vulnerable shoulders—why they ache and the best way to avoid or fix the pain... Page 220

How to choose authentic over *artificial* shoulder movements... Page 223

Why an understanding of *instinctive* human movement can help solve the shoulder pain problem... Page 224

Remove these two elements of pressing—and you will remove virtually all chronic shoulder problems... Page 225

The ultimate solution for safe, pain-free, powerful shoulders... Page 225

The mighty handstand pushup... Page 226

Using the handstand pushup to build *incredibly* powerful, muscularized shoulders in a short span of time... Page 225

How to strengthen the *vestibular system*—using handstand pushups... Page 225

8 secrets to help you perfect your all-important handstand pushup technique... Pages 228—229

Discover the ultimate shoulder and arm exercise... Page 248

Going beyond the one-arm handstand pushup... Page 252

The master of this old technique will have elbows strong as titanium axles... Page 255

The cast iron principles of Convict Conditioning success... Page 259

The missing "x factor" of training success... Page 259

The best ways to warm up... Page 260

How to create training momentum... Page 262

How to put strength in the bank... Page 263

This is the real way to get genuine, lasting strength and power gains... Page 265

Intensity—what it is and what it isn't... Page 265

Why "cycling" or "periodization" is unnecessary with bodyweight training... Page 266

How to make consistent progress... Page 266

5 powerful secrets for busting through your plateaus... Page 267

The nifty little secret of *consolidation* training... Page 268

Living by the buzzer—and the importance of regime... Page 275

5 major *Convict Conditioning* training programs... Page 276

The *New Blood* training program... Page 278

The *Good Behavior* training program... Page 279

The *Veterano* training program... Page 280

The *Solitary Confinement* training program... Page 281

The *Supermax* training program... Page 282

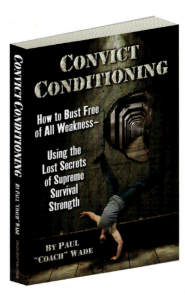

Convict Conditioning

How to Bust Free of All Weakness—Using the Lost Secrets of Supreme Survival Strength

By Paul "Coach" Wade

#B41 $39.95

eBook $19.95

The Experts Give High Praise to Convict Conditioning 2

"Coach Paul Wade has outdone himself. His first book *Convict Conditioning* is to my mind THE BEST book ever written on bodyweight conditioning. Hands down. Now, with the sequel *Convict Conditioning 2*, Coach Wade takes us even deeper into the subtle nuances of training with the ultimate resistance tool: our bodies.

In plain English, but with an amazing understanding of anatomy, physiology, kinesiology and, go figure, psychology, Coach Wade explains very simply how to work the smaller but just as important areas of the body such as the hands and forearms, neck and calves and obliques in serious functional ways.

His minimalist approach to exercise belies the complexity of his system and the deep insight into exactly how the body works and the best way to get from A to Z in the shortest time possible.

I got the best advice on how to strengthen the hard-to-reach extensors of the hand right away from this exercise Master I have ever seen. It's so simple but so completely functional I can't believe no one else has thought of it yet. Just glad he figured it out for me.

Paul teaches us how to strengthen our bodies with the simplest of movements while at the same time balancing our structures in the same way: simple exercises that work the whole body.

And just as simply as he did with his first book. His novel approach to stretching and mobility training is brilliant and fresh as well as his take on recovery and healing from injury. Sprinkled throughout the entire book are too-many-to-count insights and advice from a man who has come to his knowledge the hard way and knows exactly of what he speaks.

This book is, as was his first, an amazing journey into the history of physical culture disguised as a book on calisthenics. But the thing that Coach Wade does better than any before him is his unbelievable progressions on EVERY EXERCISE and stretch! He breaks things down and tells us EXACTLY how to proceed to get to whatever level of strength and development we want. AND gives us the exact metrics we need to know when to go to the next level.

Adding in completely practical and immediately useful insights into nutrition and the mindset necessary to deal not only with training but with life, makes this book a classic that will stand the test of time.

Bravo Coach Wade, Bravo." —**Mark Reifkind**, Master RKC, author of *Mastering the HardStyle Kettlebell Swing*

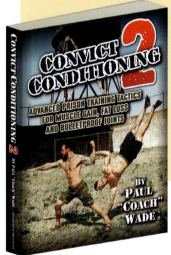

Convict Conditioning 2

Advanced Prison Training Tactics for Muscle Gain, Fat Loss and Bulletproof Joints

By Paul "Coach" Wade

#B59 **$39.95**

eBook **$19.95**

"The overriding principle of *Convict Conditioning 2* is 'little equipment-big rewards'. For the athlete in the throwing and fighting arts, the section on Lateral Chain Training, Capturing the Flag, is a unique and perhaps singular approach to training the obliques and the whole family of side muscles. This section stood out to me as ground breaking and well worth the time and energy by anyone to review and attempt to complete. Literally, this is a new approach to lateral chain training that is well beyond sidebends and suitcase deadlifts.

The author's review of passive stretching reflects the experience of many of us in the field. But, his solution might be the reason I am going to recommend this work for everyone: The Trifecta. This section covers what the author calls The Functional Triad and gives a series of simple progressions to three holds that promise to oil your joints. It's yoga for the strength athlete and supports the material one would find, for example, in Pavel's *Loaded Stretching*.

I didn't expect to like this book, but I come away from it practically insisting that everyone read it. It is a strongman book mixed with yoga mixed with street smarts. I wanted to hate it, but I love it."
—**Dan John**, author of *Don't Let Go* and co-author of *Easy Strength*

"I've been lifting weights for over 50 years and have trained in the martial arts since 1965. I've read voraciously on both subjects, and written dozens of magazine articles and many books on the subjects. This book and Wade's first, *Convict Conditioning*, are by far the most commonsense, information-packed, and result producing I've read. These books will truly change your life.

Paul Wade is a new and powerful voice in the strength and fitness arena, one that is commonsense, inspiring, and in your face. His approach to maximizing your body's potential is not the same old hackneyed material you find in every book and magazine piece that pictures steroid-bloated models screaming as they curl weights. Wade's stuff has been proven effective by hard men who don't tolerate fluff. It will work for you, too—guaranteed.

As an ex-cop, I've gone mano-y-mano with ex-cons that had clearly trained as Paul Wade suggests in his two *Convict Conditioning* books. While these guys didn't look like steroid-fueled bodybuilders (actually, there were a couple who did), all were incredibly lean, hard and powerful. Wade blows many commonly held beliefs about conditioning, strengthening, and eating out of the water and replaces them with result-producing information that won't cost you a dime."
—**Loren W. Christensen**, author of *Fighting the Pain Resistant Attacker*, and many other titles

"*Convict Conditioning* is one of the most influential books I ever got my hands on. *Convict Conditioning 2* took my training and outlook on the power of bodyweight training to the 10th degree—from strengthening the smallest muscles in a maximal manner, all the way to using bodyweight training as a means of healing injuries that pile up from over 22 years of aggressive lifting.

I've used both *Convict Conditioning* and *Convict Conditioning 2* on myself and with my athletes. Without either of these books I can easily say that these boys would not be the BEASTS they are today. Without a doubt *Convict Conditioning 2* will blow you away and inspire and educate you to take bodyweight training to a whole NEW level."
—**Zach Even-Esh**, Underground Strength Coach

Order Convict Conditioning 2 online: www.dragondoor.com/B59

24 HOURS A DAY ORDER NOW **1•800•899•5111**
Visit: www.dragondoor.com

"Paul Wade's section on developing the sides of the body in Convict Conditioning 2 is brilliant. Hardstyle!" —Pavel Tsatsouline, author of The Naked Warrior

Online Praise for Convict Conditioning 2

Best Sequel Since The Godfather 2!
"Hands down the best addition to the material on *Convict Conditioning* that could possibly be put out. I already implemented the neck bridges, calf and hand training to my weekly schedule, and as soon as my handstand pushups and leg raises are fully loaded I'll start the flags. Thank you, Coach!"
— Daniel Runkel, Rio de Janeiro, Brazil

The progressions were again sublime
"Never have I heard such in depth and yet easy to understand description of training and physical culture. A perfect complement to the first book although it has its own style keeping the best attributes of style from the first but developing it to something unique. The progressions were again sublime and designed for people at all levels of ability. The two books together can forge what will closely resemble superhuman strength and an incredible physique and yet the steps to get there are so simple and easy to understand."
—Ryan O., Nottingham, United Kingdom

Well worth the wait
"Another very interesting, and as before, opinionated book by Paul Wade. As I work through the CC1 progressions, I find it's paying off at a steady if unspectacular rate, which suits me just fine. No training injuries worth the name, convincing gains in strength. I expect the same with CC2 which rounds off CC1 with just the kind of material I was looking for. Wade and Dragon Door deserve to be highly commended for publishing these techniques. A tremendous way to train outside of the gym ecosystem." —V. R., Bangalore, India

Very Informative
"*Convict Conditioning 2* is more subversive training information in the same style as its original. It's such a great complement to the original, but also solid enough on its own. The information in this book is fantastic-- a great buy! Follow this program, and you will get stronger."
—Chris B., Thunder Bay, Canada

Just as brilliant as its predecessor!
"Just as brilliant as its predecessor! The new exercises add to the Big 6 in a keep-it-simple kind of way. Anyone who will put in the time with both of these masterpieces will be as strong as humanly possible. I especially liked the parts on grip work. To me, that alone was worth the price of the entire book."
—Timothy Stovall / Evansville, Indiana

If you liked CC1, you'll love CC2
"CC2 picks up where CC1 left off with great information about the human flag (including a version called the clutch flag, that I can actually do now), neck and forearms. I couldn't be happier with this book."
—Justin B., Atlanta, Georgia

From the almost laughably-simple to realm-of-the-gods
"*Convict Conditioning 2* is a great companion piece to the original Convict Conditioning. It helps to further build up the athlete and does deliver on phenomenal improvement with minimal equipment and space.

The grip work is probably the superstar of the book. Second, maybe, is the attention devoted to the lateral muscles with the development of the clutch- and press-flag.

Convict Conditioning 2 is more of the same - more of the systematic and methodical improvement in exercises that travel smoothly from the almost laughably-simple to realm-of-the-gods. It is a solid addition to any fitness library."
—Robert Aldrich, Chapel Hill, GA

Brilliant
"Convict Conditioning books are all the books you need in life. As Bruce Lee used to say, it's not a daily increase but a daily decrease. Same with life. Too many things can lead you down many paths, but to have Simplicity is perfect." —Brandon Lynch, London, England

Convict Conditioning 2
Advanced Prison Training Tactics for Muscle Gain, Fat Loss and Bulletproof Joints
By Paul "Coach" Wade
#B59 $39.95
eBook $19.95

Paperback 8.5 x

Mid-Level   Advanced

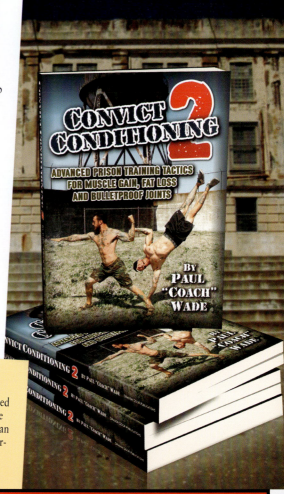

Order Convict Conditioning 2 online:
www.dragondoor.com/B59

24 HOURS A DAY ORDER NOW 1•800•899•5111
Visit: www.dragondoor.com

Go Beyond Mere "Toughness"— When You Master The Art of Bar Athletics and Sculpt the Ultimate in Upper Body Physiques

> "*Raising the Bar* is very likely the most important book on strength and conditioning to be published in the last fifty years. If you only ever get your hands on one training manual in your life, make it this one. Buy it, read it, use it. This book has the power to transform you into the ultimate bar athlete." —**Paul "Coach" Wade**, author of *Convict Conditioning*

Raising the Bar
The Definitive Guide to Bar Calisthenics
By Al Kavadlo
#B63 $39.95   eBook $19.95

1 Beginner **2** Mid-Level **3** Advanced

Raising the Bar breaks down every type of exercise you can do with a pull-up bar. From the basic two arm hang, to the mighty muscle-up, all the way to the elusive one arm pull-up, "bar master" Al Kavadlo takes you step by expert step through everything you need to do to build the chiseled frame you've always wanted.

Whether you're a die-hard calisthenics enthusiast or just looking to get in the best shape of your life, *Raising the Bar* will meet all your expectations—and then some!

The message is clear: you can earn yourself a stunning upper body with just 3 basic moves and 1 super-simple, yet amazingly versatile tool.

And what's even better, this 3 + 1 formula for upper body magnificence hides enough variety to keep you challenged and surging to new heights for a lifetime of cool moves and ever-tougher progressions!

Cast in the "concrete jungle" of urban scaffolding and graffiti-laden, blasted walls—and sourced from iconic bar-athlete destinations like Tompkins Square Park, NYC—*Raising the Bar* rears up to grab you by the throat and hurl you into an inspiring new vision of what the human body can achieve. Embrace Al Kavadlo's vision, pick up the challenge, share the Quest, follow directions—and the Holy Grail of supreme upper body fitness is yours for the taking.

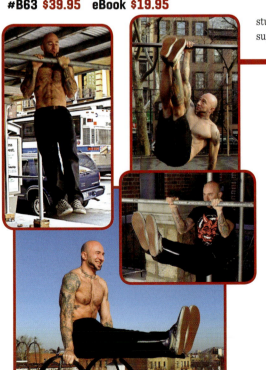

"With *Raising the Bar*, Al Kavadlo has put forth the perfect primal pull-up program. Al's progressions and demonstrations make even the most challenging exercises attainable. Anyone who is serious about pull-ups should read this book."—**Mark Sisson**, author of *The Primal Blueprint*.

A Kick Ass Encyclopedia of Bodyweight Exercises

"Al Kavadlo has put together a kick ass encyclopedia of the most powerful and most commonly used bodyweight exercises amongst the various groups of bodyweight masters.

From the most simple form of each exercise progressing to the most challenging form of each exercise, Al covers it. As a Coach and bodyweight training addict I loved all the variations shown. This book is far beyond just pull ups and there are countless exercises for upper body and abs. Al covers what is probably EVERY exercise he knows of, uses and teaches others, breaking down proper techniques, regressions and progressions. This is HUGE for the trainers out there who do NOT know how to adapt bodyweight exercises to each individual's fitness level.

If you're a fan of bodyweight training, between this book and *Convict Conditioning* you can turn your body into a deadly weapon!!!" —**Zach Even-Esh**, Manasquan, NJ

"Al has put together the companion manual for all the crazy bar calisthenics videos that you find yourself watching over and over again—a much needed resource. Within this book is a huge volume of bar exercises that will keep your pullup workouts fresh for years, and give you some insane goals to shoot for."
—**Max Shank**, Senior RKC

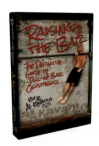

Raising the Bar
The Definitive Guide to Bar Calisthenics
DVD with Al Kavadlo
#DV090 $29.95
224 pages, 330 Photos

Order *Raising The Bar* online:
www.dragondoor.com/B63

24 HOURS A DAY ORDER NOW 1•800•899•5111
Visit: www.dragondoor.com

ANNOUNCING: Danny Kavadlo's new book,
DIAMOND-CUT ABS

HOW TO ENGINEER THE ULTIMATE SIX-PACK—MINIMALIST METHODS FOR MAXIMAL RESULTS

"*Diamond-Cut Abs* condenses decades of agonizing lessons and insight into the best book on ab-training ever written. Hands down." **—PAUL WADE**, author of **Convict Conditioning**

"Danny has done it again! *Diamond-Cut Abs* is a no-nonsense, results driven approach that delivers all the goods on abs. Nutrition, training and progression are all included, tattoos optional!" **—ROBB WOLF**, author of **The Paleo Solution**

"There are a lot of abs books and products promising a six-pack. What sets Danny's book apart is the realistic and reasonable first section of the book… His insights into nutrition are so simple and sound, there is a moment you wish this book was a stand alone dieting book." **—DAN JOHN**, author of **Never Let Go**

"Danny Kavadlo's book might be titled '*Diamond-Cut Abs*' but the truth is that it goes way BEYOND just ab training. Danny has actually created a guide to Physical Culture & LIVING healthy. The traditional fitness industry has gone astray from what the body truly needs. Since 1989, I've read a ton of abs-related books—and they don't scratch the surface of what's inside Danny's masterpiece. From powerful nutrition methods to training the entire body with a holistic approach, Diamond-Cut Abs is a vital addition to anyone's library. I LOVE it!" **—ZACH EVEN-ESH**, author of **The Encyclopedia of Underground Strength and Conditioning**

"As soon as I received *Diamond-Cut Abs*, I flipped to the table of contents. Amazingly I found what I have been fruitlessly looking for in ab books for decades: 66 pages dedicated to NUTRITION. Kavadlo passed his second Marty audition by *not* echoing all the bankrupt politically-correct, lock-step, mainstream nutritional commandments. When Dan starts riffing about eating like a horse, eating ample amounts of red meat, shellfish and the divine pig meat (along with all kinds any types of nutrient-dense food), I knew I had to give my *first ever* ab book endorsement. When he noted that he drank whiskey while getting his abs into his all time best shape, it sealed the deal for me. Oh, and the ab exercises are excellent." **—MARTY GALLAGHER**, 3-Time Powerlifting Champion, Author of **The Purposeful Primitive**

"Danny's new book definitely hits the mark. *Diamond-Cut Abs* outlines pretty much everything you'd ever need to know about building the best midsection your genetic potential allows for and without the need for any equipment. Keep up the great work, Danny!" **—BJ GADDOUR, CSCS**, author of **Men's Health Your Body is Your Barbell**, CEO of **StreamFIT.com**

"Danny flexes his expert advice in a way that's solid, applicable and often entertaining. If you want the abs of your dreams, stop looking for the quick solution everyone claims to have and get ready to learn how to maximize your efforts towards your very own set of *Diamond-Cut Abs*." **—MIKE FITCH**, creator of **Global Bodyweight Training**

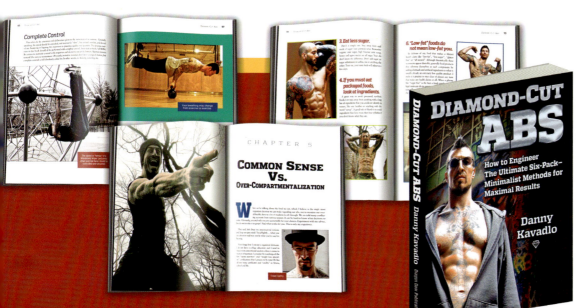

Diamond-Cut Abs

By Danny Kavadlo

Paperback 8.5 x 11
230 pages $39.95

eBook $19.95

Order *Diamond-Cut Abs* online:
www.dragondoor.com/B77

24 HOURS A DAY ORDER NOW 1•800•899•5111
Visit: www.dragondoor.com

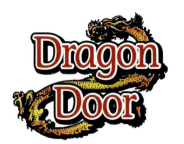

1·800·899·5111
24 HOURS A DAY • FAX YOUR ORDER (866) 280-7619
ORDERING INFORMATION

Telephone Orders For faster service you may place your orders by calling Toll Free 24 hours a day, 7 days a week, 365 days per year. When you call, please have your credit card ready.

Customer Service Questions? Please call us between 9:00am– 11:00pm EST Monday to Friday at 1-800-899-5111. Local and foreign customers call 513-346-4160 for orders and customer service

100% One-Year Risk-Free Guarantee. If you are not completely satisfied with any product—we'll be happy to give you a prompt exchange, credit, or refund, as you wish. Simply return your purchase to us, and please let us know why you were dissatisfied--it will help us to provide better products and services in the future. Shipping and handling fees are non-refundable.

Complete and mail with full payment to: Dragon Door Publications, 5 County Road B East, Suite 3, Little Canada, MN 55117

Please print clearly
Sold To: A
Name _____
Street _____
City _____
State _____ Zip _____
Day phone* _____
* Important for clarifying questions on orders

Please print clearly
Sold To: (Street address for delivery) B
Name _____
Street _____
City _____
State _____ Zip _____
Email _____

Warning to foreign customers: The Customs in your country may or may not tax or otherwise charge you an additional fee for goods you receive. Dragon Door Publications is charging you only for U.S. handling and international shipping. Dragon Door Publications is in no way responsible for any additional fees levied by Customs, the carrier or any other entity.

Item #	Qty.	Item Description	Item Price	A or B	Total

HANDLING AND SHIPPING CHARGES • NO CODS
Total Amount of Order Add (Excludes kettlebells and kettlebell kits):

$00.00 to 29.99	Add $7.00	$100.00 to 129.99	Add $14.00
$30.00 to 49.99	Add $6.00	$130.00 to 169.99	Add $16.00
$50.00 to 69.99	Add $8.00	$170.00 to 199.99	Add $18.00
$70.00 to 99.99	Add $11.00	$200.00 to 299.99	Add $20.00
		$300.00 and up	Add $24.00

Canada and Mexico add $6.00 to US charges. All other countries, flat rate, double US Charges. See Kettlebell section for Kettlebell Shipping and handling charges.

Total of Goods	
Shipping Charges	
Rush Charges	
Kettlebell Shipping Charges	
OH residents add 6.5% sales tax	
MN residents add 6.5% sales tax	

METHOD OF PAYMENT ___Check ___M.O. ___Mastercard ___Visa ___Discover ___Amex

Account No. (Please indicate all the numbers on your credit card)   EXPIRATION DATE

☐☐☐☐ ☐☐☐☐ ☐☐☐☐ ☐☐☐☐   ☐☐/☐☐

Day Phone: _____
Signature: _____ Date: _____

NOTE: We ship best method available for your delivery address. Foreign orders are sent by air. Credit card or International M.O. only. **For RUSH processing** of your order, add an additional $10.00 per address. Available on money order & charge card orders only.

Errors and omissions excepted. Prices subject to change without notice.

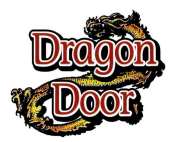

1·800·899·5111
24 HOURS A DAY • FAX YOUR ORDER (866) 280-7619
ORDERING INFORMATION

Telephone Orders For faster service you may place your orders by calling Toll Free 24 hours a day, 7 days a week, 365 days per year. When you call, please have your credit card ready.

Customer Service Questions? Please call us between 9:00am- 11:00pm EST Monday to Friday at 1-800-899-5111. Local and foreign customers call 513-346-4160 for orders and customer service

100% One-Year Risk-Free Guarantee. If you are not completely satisfied with any product—we'll be happy to give you a prompt exchange, credit, or refund, as you wish. Simply return your purchase to us, and please let us know why you were dissatisfied--it will help us to provide better products and services in the future. Shipping and handling fees are non-refundable.

Complete and mail with full payment to: Dragon Door Publications, 5 County Road B East, Suite 3, Little Canada, MN 55117

Please print clearly
Sold To: A
- Name
- Street
- City
- State _____ Zip _____
- Day phone*
- *Important for clarifying questions on orders

Please print clearly
Sold To: (Street address for delivery) B
- Name
- Street
- City
- State _____ Zip _____
- Email

Warning to foreign customers: The Customs in your country may or may not tax or otherwise charge you an additional fee for goods you receive. Dragon Door Publications is charging you only for U.S. handling and international shipping. Dragon Door Publications is in no way responsible for any additional fees levied by Customs, the carrier or any other entity.

ITEM #	QTY.	ITEM DESCRIPTION	ITEM PRICE	A OR B	TOTAL

HANDLING AND SHIPPING CHARGES • NO CODS
Total Amount of Order Add (Excludes kettlebells and kettlebell kits):

$00.00 to 29.99	Add $7.00	$100.00 to 129.99	Add $14.00
$30.00 to 49.99	Add $6.00	$130.00 to 169.99	Add $16.00
$50.00 to 69.99	Add $8.00	$170.00 to 199.99	Add $18.00
$70.00 to 99.99	Add $11.00	$200.00 to 299.99	Add $20.00
		$300.00 and up	Add $24.00

Canada and Mexico add $6.00 to US charges. All other countries, flat rate, double US Charges. See Kettlebell section for Kettlebell Shipping and handling charges.

Total of Goods	
Shipping Charges	
Rush Charges	
Kettlebell Shipping Charges	
OH residents add 6.5% sales tax	
MN residents add 6.5% sales	

METHOD OF PAYMENT ___CHECK ___M.O. ___MASTERCARD ___VISA ___DISCOVER ___AMEX

Account No. (Please indicate all the numbers on your credit card)   EXPIRATION DATE

☐☐☐☐ ☐☐☐☐ ☐☐☐☐ ☐☐☐☐   ☐☐/☐☐

Day Phone: _____

Signature: _____ Date: _____

NOTE: We ship best method available for your delivery address. Foreign orders are sent by air. Credit card or International M.O. only. **For RUSH processing** of your order, add an additional $10.00 per address. Available on money order & charge card orders only.

Errors and omissions excepted. Prices subject to change without notice.

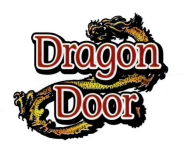

1·800·899·5111
24 HOURS A DAY • FAX YOUR ORDER (866) 280-7619
ORDERING INFORMATION

Telephone Orders For faster service you may place your orders by calling Toll Free 24 hours a day, 7 days a week, 365 days per year. When you call, please have your credit card ready.

Customer Service Questions? Please call us between 9:00am- 11:00pm EST Monday to Friday at 1-800-899-5111. Local and foreign customers call 513-346-4160 for orders and customer service

100% One-Year Risk-Free Guarantee. If you are not completely satisfied with any product—we'll be happy to give you a prompt exchange, credit, or refund, as you wish. Simply return your purchase to us, and please let us know why you were dissatisfied--it will help us to provide better products and services in the future. Shipping and handling fees are non-refundable.

Complete and mail with full payment to: Dragon Door Publications, 5 County Road B East, Suite 3, Little Canada, MN 55117

Please print clearly
Sold To: A

Name _____
Street _____
City _____
State _____ Zip _____
Day phone* _____
* Important for clarifying questions on orders

Please print clearly
Sold To: (Street address for delivery) B

Name _____
Street _____
City _____
State _____ Zip _____
Email _____

Warning to foreign customers: The Customs in your country may or may not tax or otherwise charge you an additional fee for goods you receive. Dragon Door Publications is charging you only for U.S. handling and international shipping. Dragon Door Publications is in no way responsible for any additional fees levied by Customs, the carrier or any other entity.

ITEM #	QTY.	ITEM DESCRIPTION	ITEM PRICE	A OR B	TOTAL

HANDLING AND SHIPPING CHARGES • NO CODS
Total Amount of Order Add (Excludes kettlebells and kettlebell kits):

$00.00 to 29.99 Add $7.00		$100.00 to 129.99 Add $14.00	
$30.00 to 49.99 Add $6.00		$130.00 to 169.99 Add $16.00	
$50.00 to 69.99 Add $8.00		$170.00 to 199.99 Add $18.00	
$70.00 to 99.99 Add $11.00		$200.00 to 299.99 Add $20.00	
		$300.00 and up Add $24.00	

Canada and Mexico add $6.00 to US charges. All other countries, flat rate, double US Charges. See Kettlebell section for Kettlebell Shipping and handling charges.

Total of Goods	
Shipping Charges	
Rush Charges	
Kettlebell Shipping Charges	
OH residents add 6.5% sales tax	
MN residents add 6.5% sales	

METHOD OF PAYMENT ___CHECK ___M.O. ___MASTERCARD ___VISA ___DISCOVER ___AMEX

Account No. (Please indicate all the numbers on your credit card)   EXPIRATION DATE

☐☐☐☐ ☐☐☐☐ ☐☐☐☐ ☐☐☐☐   ☐☐/☐☐

Day Phone: _____
Signature: _____   Date: _____

NOTE: We ship best method available for your delivery address. Foreign orders are sent by air. Credit card or International M.O. only. **For RUSH processing** of your order, add an additional $10.00 per address. Available on money order & charge card orders only.

Errors and omissions excepted. Prices subject to change without notice.